Reason on Trial

Reason on Trial

Keeping Human Rights in Public Health

Aden Tate

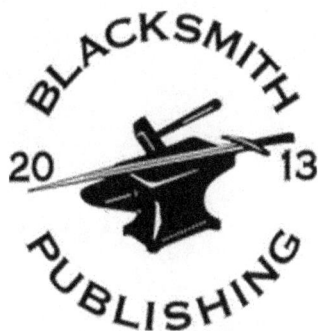

For my children and for the future generations of America who deserve to live in freedom.

Reason on Trial: Keeping Human Rights in Public Health

by Aden Tate

ISBN 9781956904093

Printed in the United States of America

Published by Blacksmith LLC
Fayetteville, North Carolina

www.BlacksmithPublishing.com

Direct inquiries and/or orders to the above web address.

Contents

Foreword

"Freedom is never more than one generation away from extinction. We didn't pass it to our children in the bloodstream. It must be fought for, protected, and handed on for them to do the same, or one day we will spend our sunset years telling our children and our children's children what it was once like in the United States where men were free." – Ronald Reagan

There is hardly an aspect of life that is not impacted by political correctness. Political correctness (PC) began as an effort to extend equality and respect to everyone. Being "PC" involves avoiding words, expressions or actions that might be perceived to exclude, marginalize, or insult particular groups of people who are disadvantaged or discriminated against. Often political correctness begins with good intentions. Ideas such as treating others the way we would like to be treated and avoiding insulting others. For example, when I was growing up in the 70s, as a general rule, one avoided discussions pertaining to race, religion or politics. There were things you simply didn't talk about in polite company. It's what you did. When such topics come up, as they often did, you were allowed to disagree. A common expression that acknowledged such a toleration in the exchange of ideas was "it's a free country." You could vote your conscience, speak your mind and hold to your own cherished notions and worldviews without the threat of being shamed, ostracized or even attacked. But, as it so often happens, the pendulum swung too far; and keeps on swinging.

Don't get me wrong here. The social justice pendulum swung in a healthy direction regarding many important issues. However, what began as an effort to extend equality and respect to everyone has now become a line that must be "toed," a slogan that must be chanted, and a mental acquiescence that must be adhered to, that is, at least if you value your job. Moreover, political correctness is highly adaptive. Things change rapidly. You have to keep up. You have to stay up on all the latest banned words, expressions or actions for fear you'll be deemed "chauvinistic," "bigoted," "patristic," or even "racist." For instance, some words that were considered PC even ten years ago are no longer tolerated. To disagree with someone, at least some people, is now considered intolerable. People get offended and triggered over words they don't like. So much so, if you trigger them, they will become physically violent and may attack you or your family and property.

What was the source of all this extreme PC business? For starters, universities have been the breeding grounds; at least in large measure. Political correctness prevents people like Ben Shapiro from speaking at certain colleges. Universities are supposed to champion the free exchange of ideas. Extreme political correctness leads to the rewriting of history so that it's in accordance with modern sensibilities. Simply put, the modern version of political correctness prevents the rational exchange of ideas and even makes us more stupid. It may even be said, I know this is a stretch (or is it?), that the movie Idiocracy was mockumentary that has become a documentary. It may be genuinely said therefore that political correctness has corrupted our institutions of higher learning to the point that they are beyond recovery.

Another source of this extreme PC business is undoubtedly the fact that Americans have become far too sensitive. In a 2016 Pew Research survey, 59% of Americans believed this to be true. Further, as the survey demonstrates, being PC is also bipartisan, not just a phenomenon on the left. And this was four years ago. To put it philosophically,

Descartes once said "I think therefore I am." It seems the expression today would be "I feel therefore I am." This is demonstrated in virtually every YouTube video where a snowflake is triggered, the facts and logic are ignored, and feelings are what carry the day. In so many of these "conversations," reason is simply not part of the exchange of ideas. Normally, the verbal interchange comes to an abrupt end when the snowflake becomes emotionally charged and begins yelling obscenities and labelling the one they disagreed with as "fascist" or "racist." Such instances remind one of George Orwell's "Thought Police" in his prescient novel 1984.

As goes the ancient axiom, "He who pays the piper calls the tune" .... which means the one who pays decides how things go. As such, political correctness has become weaponized. It's used as a tool by various social groups and especially the media who leverage it to gain moral capital and control over people's minds. Like the ferocious propaganda apparatus in Orwell's novel, Big Brother is always watching. These sycophantic suck-up talking heads genuflect to the latest Big Brother talking points. Thought crime is punished with shame. Guilt is a powerful weapon in the media's arsenal. Offenders are vilified and even called racists without any evidence. Invariably, we give ground to those who are offended about everything. Likewise, if you were to follow Big Brother's little minions long enough, one can readily note their moral flexibility. And in the end, political correctness leads to an Orwellian nightmare.

What guides any such discussion as this is values. It has been rightly said that values are like the rudder of a ship. It's small, it's below the surface but it guides the ship. Likewise, as politics are downstream from culture, the media is likened to a ship that floats along in the stream of the people, carried along with even the wildest of waves. What's the trajectory of this extreme political correctness if it's not guided by reason? The end of this PC rainbow can only be totalitarianism – prohibiting opposition on all levels of society and restricting individual freedoms. As 2020 continues to surprise us, it seems that people don't want equality, they want revenge. This is illogical as it is immoral. To cite just one rational objection: No one is alive who was a slave and one is alive who owned slaves. All of this concludes one to ask: Is this the end of the age of reason?

No discussion of this type can rightly conclude without reminding ourselves of one of the great freedoms enshrined in our Constitution – freedom of speech. "If liberty means anything at all," said George Orwell, "it means the right to tell people what they do not want to hear." Its therefore distinctively American to be okay with someone who disagrees with you. Besides, as Shakespeare once wrote, "There is nothing either good or bad, but thinking makes it so." Thus, you can become offended at anything when you're constantly looking for an offense. And so, political correctness has become the opposite of how it began. Political correctness is good to the extent where its reasonable and logical. The problem is, today's extreme political correctness is no longer about being equal, it's about being in or being out. In the series House of Cards, there's a scene that underscores this very point. Kevin Spacy says, "Welcome to the death of the age of reason. There is no right or wrong. Not anymore. There's only being in and then being out."

In light of the predicament we find ourselves in, I love this book because it sounds a clarion call for Americans to return to the foundational truths our Nation was founded on. As the author will argue, the United States, and Western civilization, was founded upon Judeo-Christian values. And if there is no Judeo-Christian foundation, then there is no United States.

This book is a timely philosophical investigation into our current national plight. Because freedom is never more than one generation away from extinction, the only thing necessary for the triumph of evil is for good men to do nothing. The incentive to read this book is it may save America.

Truth, Strength, and Honor!
Paul D. LeFavor

Preface

It was while I was in graduate school studying for my master's in public health that I first discovered the prevalence of collectivist thought within the fields of public health and healthcare. Paper after paper, textbook after textbook, all seemed to espouse the same formula for dealing with any form of public health problem whatsoever: rob people of their God-given freedoms.

As this realization dawned upon me throughout grad school it slowly turned into a state of horror as I discovered that these fellow students – these people who had likely never read the Constitution or Bill or Rights in their entire life – would soon be in positions of power over the rest of the American populace.

The arguments I both read and heard from my fellow students followed the logic of New Jersey's outlawing of soda, drastic taxes on products students didn't like, and so on. What further concerned me was that the professors never pointed out this behavior either. I cannot remember a single time throughout my entire graduate school studentship that a professor pointed out that a particular "remedy" to a "problem" would violate basic human rights. Not once did we have an in-depth discussion about Constitutional law, human rights, or anything similar. I did see some fleeting glances of this discussion in some of my textbooks, but I found the content within to be incorrect – to be arguing against human rights from a flawed foundation under the excuse of "well, it's public health, so we can do whatever we want."

And that's basically the underlying position that I learned throughout graduate school: that people believe public health is in essence a blank check – a source of unlimited power. Public health is the perfect guise for tyranny. Once one states that a particular action needs to be taken in order to "protect the public health", the greater majority of Americans seem to just roll over. Fear and superstition have taken place of the love of freedom, and thus what is thought to be security is agreed to instead.

As the years rolled by after grad school, this lesson didn't escape me, but it did slip something to the backburner of my mind. Life happened, and the importance of paying loans, paying bills, and providing for my family took the forefront, as it should have. It was with the passing of 2020 that I began to see the culmination of all the potential horrors we had discussed back in graduate years so many years ago. It seemed as if every day that I looked at the news online (for TV is no longer news, but instead propaganda.), that I was able to read about at least three new infringements on human rights by those who were in a quest to "stop the spread".

And I came to the conclusion that it was time to say something. That lesson that had been learned so long ago and that occasionally got brought up in conversation with close friends, deserved to have a broader audience. This was not because I had stumbled upon some unique truth that had been lost for all these years, but instead because freedom deserves to be defended, and this is one small way that I can be involved in the fight to keep it. To keep my mouth shut at such a time would be to be complicit in the crimes (and I do mean that in the literal sense) our politicians and their enforcement teams are committing against the American people on a daily basis.

I will not sit back silently fuming as I watch my nation (quite literally) burning. Years from now - when and if things get worse – should my children ask, "Why are things so bad today, Dad?" and I tell them why, if their next question is, "Why didn't you do anything to stop it?", I will have a response.

And this book will be a part of my proof.

1

Crafting Public Health Law

"The government big enough to give you everything you want is a government strong enough to take away everything that you have." – Rand Paul [1]

"Necessity is the plea for every infringement of human freedom. It is the argument of tyrants; it is the creed of slaves." – William Pitt, before the House of Commons, November 18, 1783 [2]

Anybody who works in the field of government policy creation – or even government policy advocacy – needs to understand that they are first and foremost civil *servants*. One does not *rightfully* take a government office for the riches and powers that it bestows on individuals. One rightfully takes a government office *only if* they are truly wanting to make a positive difference on their countrymen. The mindset of George Washington should be the mindset of every American in office – that of a man who is willing to answer the call of his people, but who is more than willing – in fact, even *desires* – to voluntarily give up power and return to a quieter life.

To argue for a nation to *not* possess people within its boundaries who are envious of power solely for power's sake is to hope for utopia. Such will never happen on this present earth. Mankind is fallen, and until one understands that –

1

that mankind is *not* inherently good, but instead inherently wicked – then they will continue to hope in vain for utopian ideals. This is not to say that it is wrong to be idealistic, or even that we should not put good and just laws into place, but instead to say that we *have* to anticipate that there are going to be evil men who will at some time or another weasel their way into government positions of power.

That all being said, one of the foundations of the character of the best public health policy creator is that they don't desire power for power's sake.

The next thing that those in positions of government need to understand is that "the purpose of law and of government is the protection of individual rights."[3] Far too many American citizens today are completely illiterate when it comes to Americanism, the philosophy behind freedom and human rights, capitalism, and the US Constitution. It is because of this (in large part brought about by the abysmal failure known as our public school system and public universities) - for evidence of why I hold such a belief read about the communist infiltration in *None Dare Call It Treason*, examine Common Core, the 1619 Project, critical race theory, or any of the other nonsensical garbage that our school system is teaching our children today - that the average American has absolutely no idea what the ultimate goal of government is or why government is created in the first place.

Americans as a whole now believe that if a government makes a law, then it automatically must be obeyed and followed, and that their government rightfully has the power to push through quite literally anything it can imagine into becoming both law and policy.[1] However, as defender of liberty Frederic Bastiat astutely pointed out, law does not necessarily equal justice. There are a host of laws created that are in fact quite the opposite: the rubber stamp of approval on theft, kidnapping, and murder. If you have a graduate student who is currently working on their master's in public health administration – a student who is being trained to work in the field of public health policy creation – and they already have this ill-formed notion that governments can do whatever they want – when they get into a position of power to make public health policy, guess what they will do?

They will believe that they have the ultimate power over the rest of the populace – their friends, families, and neighbors – anytime something is being discussed within the bounds of public health. If they don't like the idea of your eating fast food three times a week, they may believe that they have the right to keep you from ever doing such in the first place.

Their misconceived notion that they have total power – their misunderstanding of why governments are created by men in the first place – to protect individual rights – will lead to their becoming yet another petty tyrant bent on controlling and forcing people to *their* will. And if the people won't comply with this newly created tyrant's every whim – if they decide that they *like* eating fast food three times a week – let it be remembered that tyrants always resort to increasing levels of force to get their will to be followed. Whether that comes in the form of hefty fines, imprisonment, confiscation of property, or worse, a tyrant always utilizes men with guns to accomplish his (evil) will.

Before going any further though, it is very important that we take a closer look at the foundations of crafting public health law. There are undoubtedly going to be some situations in which something has to be done to protect the health of a nation. However, as we've pointed out, it's typically the case that those who craft such laws have little to no understanding of what it means to be an American, freedom, or what exactly is written within the Bill of Rights. More often than not, I've noticed that those who craft public health law believe that they *have* powers that in reality they do *not*. However, it's often not realized by an ill-informed public that their rights are being infringed by one who truly has no power to create such a law in the first place.

For any novice public health policy maker, there are a number of foundational truths that need to be kept in mind throughout the entire process of policy creation. The question going into any policy creation meeting does not need to be "what's the quickest way to get the result that we want?" but instead, "what's the best way to get the result that we need *without violating human rights in the process?*"

As Ayn Rand said, "Potentially, a government is the most dangerous threat to man's rights..."[4] This meshes hand in hand with what George Washington had to say when he stated that government, like fire, can be a useful tool, but a fearful master. [The full statement is this: "Government is not reason; it is not eloquence; it is force! Like fire, it is a dangerous servant and a fearful master."][5]

Perhaps it would be best to start off by looking at what the proper role of governments are in the first place. In my observation, I've noticed that virtually nobody within public health roles can accurately name what the end goals of just governments are to be. Americans are becoming progressively stupider than they've ever been before, and I've yet to find a public health program out there that requires the students to truly delve deeply into studying the philosophy of law, of government, of human rights, and of freedom. This is truly a scary thought when you consider that these are the very students who will soon become responsible for decisions which affect law, government, human rights, and freedom.

So at the very basic level, what is it that these students need to know? I believe that it would be wise to look once more to what Ayn Rand has to say. "Since the protection of individual rights is the only proper purpose of a government, it is the only proper subject of legislation: all laws must be based on individual rights and aimed at their protection."[6]

This above quote needs to especially be kept in mind when it comes to crafting public health law. Public health is the perfect guise for tyranny, and those who forget this will one day discover what a nightmare world they live in when public health officials are given a blank check. Imagine a world where it has been deemed a health risk to go to church, have certain political beliefs, pray, have more than one child, and the like. Likely, not much imagination is needed. Those who are reading through this book now have lived through such a world. But just know that despite the terror that was 2020-2021, things could always be worse. That's why a proper understanding of how to mesh human rights with public health is essential.

In order to avoid such a nightmare world, crafters of public health law need to know that "the proper functions of a government fall into three broad categories, all of them involving the issues of physical force and the protection of men's rights: *the police*, to protect men from criminals – *the armed services*, to protect men from foreign invaders – *the law courts*, to settle disputes among men according to objective laws."[7]

What needs to be remembered is that it is *force* that gives a government leverage. For every law that is crafted, whether that be within the field of public health or not, government rubber stamps the use of physical force against those who won't comply. One could argue that they aren't going to send the police after somebody, but instead are going to give a hefty fine, force them to attend a food safety class, or threaten to pull their business license, but remember that if the "criminal" decides that they're not going to comply with *that* punishment, the next step is going to involve sending men with guns, batons, and handcuffs – men with the ability to throw one in a prison full of 300 pound sodomites - to the scene to physically enforce compliance.

Thus, the stricter the law, the more likely and more often one is going to have to resort to physical force to get the law to be complied with. This can rapidly result in a downward spiral towards a police state being created.

"But I'm trying to *help!*" the public health official proclaims. "I'm trying to protect the public *health!*" Let us not forget that it is not the road to Heaven that is paved with good intentions. As F.A. Hayek stated in *The Road to Serfdom* (a book which should be required reading for all public health students), "...in Germany it was largely people of good will, men who were admired and held up as models in the democratic countries, who prepared the way for, if they did not actually create, the forces which now stand for everything they detest."[8]

Everybody wants to believe that they are the hero. One of the key ways to ensure that one is not actually becoming the villain however, is to look at the means by which they are attempting to secure their goals. Nobody wants to be labeled a Nazi. Those were absolutely terrible people, responsible for absolutely heinous crimes. Yet, as FA Hayek says, "...many who think themselves infinitely superior to the aberrations of Naziism, and sincerely hate all its manifestations, work at the same time for ideals whose realization would lead straight to the abhorred tyranny."[8]

This is done by the advocating and pushing for policies that infringe upon human rights and human freedom. If we imagine collectivism and tyranny as an impenetrable concrete wall with Lady Liberty on one side of it, every time that these tyrannical policies are advocated for – even by those who on the surface would say that Nazi Germany and Soviet Russia were terrible places – they are (perhaps) unwittingly pushing that concrete wall even closer on Lady Liberty's turf. It is only a matter of time after a consistent number of these laws have been approved that she will helplessly fall off the cliff.

Thus, it is absolutely vital that anybody involved with the creation of public health policy be well-versed in what it means to be free. To be a seasoned lover of liberty. To have otherwise in office is to have nothing more than a smiling time bomb.

The Final Steps of Public Health Law Creation

Once it has been determined that a particular new public health law *does* actually need to be passed and put into effect – that it will not violate individual human rights and will accomplish its goal with minimal problems – then it is absolutely vital that the law is worded within the legislature in as explicit as a manner as possible. There should be no guesswork to what the law means whatsoever. There should be no ill-defined broad terms used within the law whatsoever. It is in part because of such ill-defined laws that government overreach is able to grow. As FA Hayek says, "...the discretion left to the executive organs wielding coercive power should be reduced as much as possible..."[9]

This is absolutely vital to keeping a small and controllable government from growing into a monster that controls its people. History has proven that unless one explicitly states what the government can and cannot do the power of government will quickly grown into a totalitarian state. True, even when one *does* explicitly state government restrictions (such as with the Bill of Rights) totalitarianism seems to be the natural progress of things (as evidenced within the history of America, from its birth of freedom in 1776 to the continued decline into slavery [in full by 2020] at an incredibly rapid pace roughly beginning around the time of F.D. Roosevelt.)

Very explicit instructions must be made leaving as little wiggle room and room for interpretation as possible. Though "interpretation" is never to be a part of the judicial system – it is solely a role of enforcing the law as created by the legislative branch – history has once more proven that over time this form of entropy will only grow in prevalence. The best we can do is to slow the process down exponentially, and to provide the people the means necessary to change their government for the better as the time comes.

2

Privacy

"The right of the people to be secure in their persons, houses, papers, and effects, against unreasonable searches and seizures, shall not be violated, and no Warrants shall issue, but upon probable cause, supported by Oath or affirmation, and particularly describing the place to be searched, and the persons or things to be seized."
– The Fourth Amendment of the Bill of Rights

Privacy is foundational to a free society. It is the abolition of privacy that assists in the growth of a totalitarian state. When privacy is stolen from citizens by the government, the seedling of absolute power is watered and flourishes. Who can argue for the benefits of an all-knowing government? History has proven that politicians are very much capable of rapidly changing their minds on both what is legal and what is not. Within the United States there are a plethora of examples of such. We can find countless instances of where items such as bump stocks, AR-15s, 30-round magazines, certain medications, particular fertilizers, particular firearms and so on are perfectly legal one day, and within the span of 24 hours all holders of such items are now felons and deemed to be a danger to society. As a result, the strictest of punishments should await them, and they should no longer be deemed eligible to vote for the leaders within their society.

We can see this with actions as well. One day working within a particular field, installing certain parts to an engine, using a particular form of chemical and so on is perfectly legal, and within the span of 24 hours it becomes illegal to do so entirely or without hefty licensing fees and certifications. As a locksmith, I've witnessed this firsthand. I've seen men and women who were absolutely free to provide for their families in their chosen profession for years. Then, all of a sudden, a law has been passed, and unless those very same people now pay substantial fees, attend certain classes, register, and go through the hoops to be granted the newly created locksmith's license, they are operating illegally.

When locksmiths resisted this order, refusing to go through this red tape and pay these fees/taxes, armed men showed up to their businesses and *closed their business*, forcing them to comply or else risk not being able to feed their families, pay their mortgages, and so on. This was all for a occupation that had been free to enter for decades past. When politicians change their mind, making certain occupations or actions illegal, they always send men with guns to enforce their whims on the populace.

Beliefs are not immune to such government mind-changing either. What was once considered to be common knowledge (such as the wickedness of homosexuality/pedophilia/etc.) can be turned into a hate crime to speak of or act on within the span of a number of hours. Just look at the policies throughout many European nations where police officers refuse to enter refugee strongholds in the cities where the rape statistics of skyrocketed, but those very same officers are more than willing to lock up a respectable native businessman because he's said something that's been deemed to be a hate crime.

Chapter 2 – Privacy

Even one's genetic makeup can quickly become illegal as the Jews of 1930s Germany quickly discovered. It was solely because of their heritage that they were labeled as fit for extermination in the literal sense. Numerous other nations throughout history have demonstrated this same truth through the use of government mandated genocide. Whether we're talking about the Armenian genocide, China's war against Uighurs, or what have you, the point can very easily be seen that sometimes your DNA structure can be used as an argument to murder you.

And though one may argue that "if you have nothing to hide, you have nothing to fear" the fact remains that such an argument is a collection of utter nonsense. Those who tout such theories are often to be found with curtains on their windows, clothes on their privates, and doors on their bedrooms. They would probably object to your rooting through their nightstands. But if they have nothing to hide, why do they feel the need to hide things? It is because they have an inherent understanding of the value and importance of privacy. Without it, we would all live in the glass houses of Zamyatin's dystopian novel *We*.

This basic understanding of how foundational privacy is to freedom is built into the American understanding of life and the Constitution. It was this understanding that caused the Founding Fathers to incorporate protection from unwarranted search and seizure by police and other governing authorities into our founding documents. This is in part to protect one's personal privacy.

The repeated argument that one will hear against privacy though is that it is not safe. It is generally those who are fearful of some happenstance who argue the strongest for the stripping of others privacy. For example, we saw after 9/11 George Bush's incorporation of the Patriot Act, something which was created with the intention of stopping terrorism (a rather vague term), and did so by robbing the entire American people of their privacy, as Edward Snowden later revealed. This was all deemed to be in the service of the public good – to protect others' safety – and thus, justified.

Within the span of public health, we see the same argument being used over and over again. There's no situation within American health that better demonstrates this argument against the privacy of others due to the fear for one's own safety than the 2020 coronavirus panic. There can be no doubt that in some situations it is beneficial for the government to have an idea of what the scope of a particular disease, condition, or infection is. Nobody has a problem with bubonic plague being a reportable disease within the United States. Should you end up infected with the plague (Which *does* still happen. To my knowledge the most recent case took place around Lake Tahoe in 2020.), your case will be reported to the federal government.[1]

However, there is a vast difference in anonymous health data being reported to the government and being hunted down and tracked to in order to report an expansive breadth of data to the government. I am not aware of any reasoning that is given for invading one's privacy that is more often used than the excuse of "security". Privacy must be invaded or voided so that we can all be "safe", we are told. What exactly we are told we are being kept safe from changes based on the situation, but the argument cannot be successfully made unless a fair amount of fear has already been generated – whether well-founded or not.

Always Watching

Is the idea of being watched 24/7 by some other human concerning to you? Is the very thought not rather disturbing? The idea of such brings thoughts of George Orwell's *1984* to mind. It's *because* people do not want to always be watched that street cameras have been such a contentious issue. Is it not an invasion of privacy to have a camera on every street corner throughout the city? Does the possession of that much data not lead to an incredible amount of power that no man (or organization) should hold? As Lord Acton stated, "Absolute power corrupts absolutely."

When New York places 500,000 smart streetlights throughout the state – all hooked up to the Internet of Things, something long associated with a high vulnerability of being hacked – should we not be concerned? Smart Cities Dive, the creators of such technology, stated that the tech "can then be upgraded to have sensors with features like environmental monitoring and noise detection." Is it too far to think that recording conversations could be a feature of "noise detection"? Smart Cities Dive goes on to note that these smart streetlights can be used to monitor large gatherings "in a bid to try and prevent the spread of infection [of coronavirus]".[2] Is this not Big Brother at work? When your own city surrounds you with cameras and audio recording equipment, you should be concerned.

There is most certainly something to be said about thermal imaging as well. HIPAA – one of the greatest pieces of legislation (at least at its ideological roots) passed within the US – stated that individuals have the right for their own personal health information to be protected. No longer could your nurse go and tell all of her friends at book club about your anal fissure, STD, bariatric surgery, or the like. HIPAA was a validation of the fact that people have a right to their own privacy, and that others do *not* have the right to invade it. Nobody within the medical field can go around telling others your medical history, medical conditions, or anatomical measurements and data points unless they have your express permission due to HIPAA.

That being said, why do others think they have the right to your *temperature* data? Should such not be protected under HIPAA as well? I believe it is.

It's often not even as if people will ask to take your temperature (though this is very common throughout the world at the moment). In many cases, your temperature is being taken without your knowledge through the use of artificial intelligence. Is this not an invasion of privacy? Is it not a violation of HIPAA?

Let's follow this act to its logical conclusions. What would happen if we discovered that we could chart peoples' pheromone levels to determine if they were sick with a contagious illness or not? What if some new form of respiratory illness sent your pheromone levels sky-high, causing the opposite sex to have an intense desire to be in close proximity to you? Would we then force people to give us their pheromone information? What if we discover that a certain temperature pattern is common for a contagious disease? As a result, we engage in whole body temperature scanning of people as they walk in a room. We can now see who is sweating profusely from their crotch and armpits. We now know who has a butt sweat problem. Is that not an invasion of your privacy? And don't think that such may not be happening already. Many buildings throughout the states – including my own work site – currently utilize Smart Pass technology.

Smart Pass is a facial recognition tech that eliminates the need for manual temperatures. You simply look into the screen, and it records who you are and reads your thermal information – decreeing if you are a safe person to be around or not.[3]

Perchance you have seen the hit TV series *Person of Interest*. Within this series, one of the main characters has created a super-intelligence that is connected to the video and audio feeds of every camera in the country. It is created with the purpose of stopping terrorism. It sees everything, feeds all that data into an algorithm, and then is able to determine who is likely to engage in a criminal act. In some ways, it's very similar to the film *Minority Report*, in which a trio of humans connected to a machine are able to predict crime before it actually occurs. Privacy is destroyed in both cases, and determinism – the idea of fate fully controlling one's actions with there being no possibility of free will – are the outcomes. Though in both series crime and terrorism drop drastically, the question remains: are these worlds that we would want to live in? Both stories point out the terrors and intricacies of why we should not. If we eliminate the concept of free will even existing, we can justify any level of evil simply because a person engages in certain activities (e.g. skeet shooting), likes certain types of music (e.g. acid rock), or believes certain ideals (e.g. libertarianism) solely because they are variables within our crime-predicting algorithm we believe are predictors of future criminal actions.

In what was possibly the only wise decision that the city of Portland has ever made, the city council there voted unanimously to ban government use of facial recognition within the city. This came shortly after it was revealed/leaked(?) that the federal government had compiled the entirety of America's driver's license photos into a massive facial recognition database. This technology has given the government the capability to track people in real-time. If somebody from the government wants to know where you are, they now have a *very* good chance of finding you.

For students of history, this should terrify you. The worst kind of prisoner to be is a political prisoner. If you tick off the wrong person in office, you could very easily end up being on somebody's *literal* watch-list. The consequences of such can be severe. Humans are fallible, fickle, easily angered, hold grudges, commonly irrational, and potentially vindictive as well. Why trust your well-being to such? Why give one the power to know where they could hurt you at any given time?[4]

For example, just look at New Jersey Governor Chris Christie. His office was shown to have *caused* massive traffic jams *on purpose* as a form of political payback to a nearby mayor.[5] What could be the consequences of such? People not able to get to the ER in time? People missing weddings, funerals, important doctor visits that could not be replaced? Imagine the power that is necessitated to cause traffic jams, and then actually having the ability to do so! People have abused the system before – arguably every system ever made. To think that such would not occur with widespread Big Brother systems is to be willfully stupid or incredibly naïve.

To return to our argument against the violation of our health privacy though, what do you do when your school district requires you to wear a Bluetooth armband to monitor your temperature? This has actually happened within the US during 2020.[6]

This is rather concerning when you consider that FitBits and other heartrate monitoring wristbands have been found capable of determining when you are having sex or not.[7] When data scientists look at the data and see a massive spike in your heart rate at 2AM, they probably have a good idea of what it is that you're doing. Does a taxpayer-funded government-run institution have the right to extract such information from you? If they can force you to do this, what else can they force you to do? Keep in mind that if you choose to not go to school because of such, you can quickly end up in a prison cell. While one university is one thing, what happens when public schools across the board decide to engage in such mandatory technology?

What happens if you don't have the time or resources to pull your child out of public school when such is mandated? You're stuck! If you don't send your child to the state-sponsored school, you risk the state kidnapping your child from you. Yet the state has now created a policy which violates privacy! It becomes a rather dangerous slippery slope to tread upon, does it not?

Your child's school has been turned into yet *another* source of government intrusion as well. Within the book *1984*, every citizen has a TV-camera within their home that constantly monitors their actions. We now have such with virtual learning. As your child attends their virtual classroom, you now have a government employee getting access to what the inside of your home looks like – with the expected, terrifying results. For many parents, the very idea of the concept of Child Protective Services terrifies them, especially given the state of modern society. People have grown more unattached from logic, more emotionally driven, and as a result, we have all heard the horror stories about how social services was called on a perfectly normal family and their children were marched off to foster care as a result.

In Colorado, 12-year-old Isaiah Elliot was taking an online art class when he flashed a toy gun across his computer screen. He was promptly suspended, and then reported *to police*, who then conducted a welfare check on the child. The underlying philosophy here is either: A) little boys with toy guns are apparently dangerous, or; B) the police obviously need to intervene in the situation because it is *apparent* that his parents are not taking care of him. After all, they let him play with a *toy gun*. Forget the fact that I can virtually guarantee you those cops play with toy guns with their sons.

If such is the case – that toy guns are inherently dangerous, and that little boys should not be playing with them - shouldn't Nerf be outlawed? Yet we permit constant commercials for Nerf guns on every children's' TV channel out there, it seems. Where is the consistency? It's wrong to have a toy gun, but it's ok to have a toy gun? Does this not make any sense to anybody else?

This wasn't an isolated incident either. A similar case took place in Maryland, where an 11-year-old boy had the police called on him because a teacher spotted a *BB gun* hanging on his bedroom wall during a Google Meet class on his laptop. He was *in his own home* (where BB guns are allowed), and didn't even touch the thing, but apparently its very presence was enough of a sign of some severe mental illness that the boy needed to be attended to by the police.[8]

And in other nations, it's even worse. Africa – a continent that is not particularly known for its defense of human rights – has created what's called PanaBIOS (technically, the African Union has, but I digress). PanaBIOS is a biosurveillance tech for COVID. Out of the entire continent of Africa – out of all 54 countries there – only 27 actually have fully functioning privacy and data protection laws. Ghana in particular seems to have let their understanding of privacy fall by the wayside. New legislation there gives their president "emergency powers" which enable him to "fight COVID" by mining data from Ghana's citizens' phone data.

With this new legislation the president can literally order telecom companies to turn over the information on a customer's subscriber database, mobile money merchant codes, address, uncashed subscriber mobile money transfer data, and subscriber cell reference data.[9] You can probably already imagine the hidden dangers here.

"Papers, please."

When freedom of movement is completely restricted, you no longer live in a free society. As others have mentioned, you don't necessarily have to restrict movement or an action in the traditional sense either in order to violate someone's freedom. It's not necessarily roadblocks throughout every major road that are utilized to violate freedom of movement (though that has been done in the name of public health as well). You can just as easily utilize *other* ways to restrict movement of a free people. One of the chief ways to do such is through the requirements of documents to go anywhere.

England – a modern slave-state – has demonstrated such in their (stated) quest for public health. As of September of 2020, they were planning a new digital ID card for all of their subjects. The online ID has the ability to be used for "daily activities" such as proving your age, registering with your general practitioner, and buying properties from a different location.[10]

They went further in November of 2020. It was then that the Behavioral Insights Team (BIT) – a group of British government advisors specializing in human behavior - began suggesting that people be given COVID wristbands after they had tested negative for COVID-19. These wristbands would then *allow* them to travel and enter venues, while those who refused to be tested, or tested positive, would continue to be under draconian lockdown laws. The BIT put out a report stating that Slovakia had gotten things right with having 97% of the citizens complying with mandatory COVID testing. Thus, the rest of the world should fall in line too, I suppose, right?

What the BIT *didn't* state however, was that Slovakians *had* to comply because their health authorities told them that they would continue to be subject to curfews and lockdowns should they not. The 97% who did comply were given paper certificates they had to carry around with them on their person or they risked police harassment.[11] I would argue that a nation with such a tangled history with Russian troop presence likely has some ingrained memory that makes them fearful to go against what the government has mandated as well.

The government of the US - "the land of the free" - is no better when it comes to such tyrannical restrictions and invasions of privacy. On December 2, 2020, the Department of Defense released images of what it claims to be the new vaccination record card and vaccination kits that they were going to begin sending out at some point in the very near future. According to Dr. Kelly Moore, associate director of the Immunization Action Coalition, "Everyone will be issued a written card that they can put in their wallet that will tell them what they had and when their next dose is due." She went on to say, "Let's do the simple, easy thing first. Everyone's going to get that."[12]

As Moore has stated, the issuing of a vaccination card is only a first step. Such a piece of paperwork can very easily be turned into a government issued permission slip to use public transit, travel to other states within the Union, or enter government offices. If the issuance of such a government ID is the easy thing, then what on earth could be some of the more *difficult* problems that Moore is alluding to? Mandatory vaccination? Seizure of assets for the non-compliant? Only the future will tell.

Coronavirus vaccination clinics will also report their state immunization registries with the new DOD paperwork regarding which vaccine was given. This way third parties will be able to verify the truthfulness of vaccine cards. Is that not rather alarming as well? Not only is a form of government ID being issued to you, but they are making it as difficult as possible to fool the system with it. And has anyone wondered whether the state has any right to your personal vaccination history to begin with? Is that not an invasion of your right to medical privacy? Is it not a violation of HIPAA?

The push for some form of ID for vaccination grew to terrifying heights throughout 2019-2021. It was within this time frame that the Bill and Melinda Gates Foundation funded research for a team of MIT researchers to develop an ink that could be embedded in the skin alongside of a vaccine itself, creating what is called a "quantum dot tattoo". This tattoo can only be seen via a special smartphone camera app and filter. That ink itself is comprised of specialized tiny semiconducting crystal that reflect light and glow when exposed to infrared light. The project allegedly came about following a direct request from Bill Gates himself.[13]

When we get to a point in society where we are branding those who have received a vaccine, we are setting the stage for medical apartheid. We now have visible proof of who has obeyed with the health mandates that those in power have issued, and consequentially, we have visible proof of those who have not. Of those who have disagreed with our mandates for whatever reason has seemed viable to them. Whether they disagree due to safety concerns, religious reasons, or just for the principle of the matter, a vaccine tattoo is nothing more than the modernization of a yellow star being sewn onto somebody's shirt.

Now that 2021 is upon us, the push for a vaccine passport seems to have reached full steam with public health officials loudly proclaiming during interviews that such is what's needed in order to get "back to normal". Even Joe Biden could be found on TV saying that Americans are down to two choices: either wear a mask or get the shot. To say such is to argue for the necessity of a vaccine passport in the first place, for how else are you going to determine if the correct people are masked or not?

As such, it seems that it is a very clear US policy for a vaccine passport to be instituted on a national scale. A good question to ask however, is whether or not anybody within a public health setting has any right to mandate or enforce such in the first place.

We've already covered how a nation that institutes special passports to block movement within the nation is not a nation of free men. The Founding Fathers of American took it as a basic supposition that free movement was inherent to freedom. They would have never dreamed that there would have been people blatantly stupid enough to decree that you could still be free without having freedom of movement.

For example, one needs look no further than New York City. As of August 2020, they've set up checkpoints throughout many of the city's entry points, where all are stopped and asked a series of questions about their recent travel history. What states you've recently been to, when, the address you're traveling from, how long you plan to be at a certain location, what your primary mode of travel will be, if children are coming with you, and your contact info are all collected.[14] Is this an example of a free society?

To examine such, think of a person who has been placed on house arrest. They're "free" to go about their daily business, but does anybody in their right mind have any misconceptions as to whether or not that man is free? By no means! He's a prisoner of his own house! To craft a vaccine passport in order to restrict movement from state to state is to make a man a prisoner of his own state, town, city, or whatever other geographic unit of measurement that you would like to use. It's to place a man in a different form of house arrest.

What about the usage of a vaccine passport for other purposes though? What about using it as necessary proof to enter a church, business, restaurant, or any other building? To argue for such is to craft a massive invasion of privacy into the very fabric of being an American. It's to say that unless you comply with the official government standpoint on the issue of COVID-19 (or any other infectious agent, for that matter) you will be treated as a second-class citizen, only capable of visiting certain venues, and resultingly being placed in a state of house arrest once more.

Can it be said that the man who is *not allowed* to enter a restaurant with friends, to attend a parent-teacher conference, to shop for his own groceries, or to go to a concert without having the necessary vaccine passport is under any other domain than that of house arrest? He's not allowed to go anywhere! A vaccine passport thus restricts freedom of movement as well as restricts freedom to do business and is not a friend to lovers of freedom anywhere on earth. What is next? Do we start having different entrances to buildings for the vaxxed and unvaxxed much akin to the race segregation that we had back in the 1960s? Because make no mistake, that *is* what's being argued for.

To argue for the mandate of a vaccine passport is to argue that we need Gestapo agents to stand at every corner demanding those they come into contact with to "State your name and race." While perhaps it may not exactly be one's race that is being searched for now, you're political, scientific, and possibly even religious beliefs are now being called into question for the public record anytime that you go out into public, and this *always* results in a very scary outcome in the near future.

A Cashless Society

Cash is truly one of the last bastions of privacy, and therefore freedom. As soon as cash disappears - as soon as electronic payments become mandatory – whether through government intervention or through private parties no longer accepting cash – then you have witnessed your country take one step closer to the creation of a totalitarian state.

Though there has been a war on cash for years, it was throughout the year 2020 that we saw new fuel being added to the anti-cash war. Cash was deemed to be dirty and a vector of disease. CNN berated people for using cash with headlines such as "Do NOT take a bunch of cash out of the bank" and "Dirty money: the case against using cash during the coronavirus outbreak". People in turn became afraid to use it, setting aside one of the most important protectors of their freedom in favor of cleaner and "safer" electronic payments.[15]

The New York times found that the 2020 coronavirus situation was indeed propelling the US towards a cashless society. And the US is not alone on the matter. India, Kenya, Sweden, and the UN all promoted cashless payments in the name of public health throughout 2020 as well. Valdis Dombrovskis, the European Commission vice president for financial services, publicly stated that it was "time to swap your coins for payment cards – safer for containing coronavirus." Why anyone would want to listen to authorities such as the UN who are known for their human rights violations is absolutely beyond me, but the fact of the matter is that people listened.

Within Italy, the volume of e-commerce surged more than 80% throughout 2020, compared to prior years. This, on a continent that *prior* to covid, used cash for 80% of its transactions. And all of this despite the fact that there is *no* medical evidence that cash transmits covid-19.[16]

So, why the push? Why do we end up with bankers such as Brian Moynihan, CEO of Bank of America saying, "We want a cashless society"?[14] Why do governments push a cashless society? The reason has to do with the data it gives them into your personal life. To have a society that does not have cash – that solely relies upon electronic forms of payment – is to have a society that can fully be tracked. Every purchase you make, whether that be for guns, ammo, body armor, smoke grenades, fertilizer, sodas, cigarettes, alcohol, condoms – *everything* – can then be tracked by the government. They know what you are buying, how much of it you are buying, and where you are getting it from. It is one of the most complete invasions of privacy that there can be.

Venezuela – a prime example of a totalitarian state – banned all cash entirely during 2020. Only electronic payments are currently accepted there. I would argue that one of the main reasons that they pushed this through was to flatten the black market there. If there is a black market, you no longer have complete control. If you have totalitarian policies, they do not work if they cannot be enforced with a sledgehammer. All forms of dissent must be completely crushed. And is there any wonder that there is a black market in a country where four rolls of toilet paper go for $21.02 USD, a small stick of butter goes for $15.01 USD, and 18 eggs go for $35.05?[17]

If you can't afford such prices for daily essentials (and nobody can in Venezuela. The people there have been pushed into poverty by socialism), then you resort to bartering. You resort to alternate forms of payment. You find ways to work around the system. However, given that any of these methods negates the complete control, I don't think that it will be long before rather drastic punishments are meted out against those who are found engaging in such forms of commerce. Any failures of the socialist system are never blamed on socialism itself, but instead on a convenient scapegoat. Black market shoppers make a very good one within socialism.

Such prices are the very nature of government economic intervention. They *create* poverty. They create famine. They create illness. They create death. History has given us countless examples of such. And yet, we are still pushing for the same policy of a cashless society here in the United States, whether that once again be through government intervention or business policy. In July 2020, the Federal

Reserve unveiled their new concept of the "Fedcoin", a federally managed alternative to bitcoin and other cryptocurrencies.

The first thing that one needs to understand about cryptocurrencies is that the idea was created by a libertarian who sought a way to further protect the privacy of the individual against government intrusion. As such, governments have done their best to destroy it – yet it *currently* has gained enough popularity that it seems to be safely embedded within pop culture at the moment.

In the meantime, the Fedcoin is being touted as a means to provide a universal basic income to Americans. The Federal Reserve would both create and maintain the account of every American, and who is buying what and why could easily be extrapolated by data scientists, algorithms, or artificial intelligences. Goods and services that politicians have then deemed to be unfavorable could be better controlled.[14,18]

Even at the private level, cashless societies are being pushed. Throughout 2020 we were told that there was a national coin shortage. Whether this was due to new coins not being minted, or due to people having to spend all of their money at home (due to lockdowns) is disputable, but the fact remains that a lot of people had a difficult time finding appropriate coinage throughout the year. It got to the point that some companies even refused to give change back. CVS, Kroger, and Walmart all began *refusing* to give change at some locations. They decided that instead of giving you your money back to make purchases of your own choosing (e.g. electric bills/car payments/mortgages) that they would either donate the money to a charity of your own choice, or instead give you the money back in store credit.[6]

Is this nothing more than a veiled form of theft? "We're sorry, sir. We know it's *your* money. We know you paid us with legal tender. But we simply will not give you back the legal tender that is *due* to you. We are going to take the money that we owe you, and then we're going to give it to a charity that *we* personally approve of."

And don't think that electronic payments being denied for products that are not approved by pop culture is a conspiracy theory either. It's already been put into practice. Capital One, Visa, and Paypal are but a few of the "pay giants" that have refused to process payments for products they deem to be short of their morality standards.[20] And this isn't for actual immoral objects either. One can still easily purchase pornography – as much as you want – via any of these payment methods. This limit on purchases is typically used against those who are supporters of the Second Amendment – against those who want to purchase guns, ammo, or other firearm accoutrements.

These companies have decided that you shouldn't be able to purchase those products. And how do they do this? By monitoring what you are buying. By knowing who you want to pay. If either what you are purchasing, or who you are purchasing from are on the company's blacklist, then you will have your payment denied, as it will not process. While there are ways to work around this problem (such as masked debit cards via Privacy.com that will disguise both what you are purchasing and from who), the point is that this is tangible proof of the argument I've been trying to make here.

When you take away anonymity from purchases – when there is some Overseer that gets to see what you're buying – they very well may decide that they don't like you buying what you're buying and prevent you from doing so. Farfetched? Nope. It's happening as we speak.

Drones

I am most certainly not anti-technology. I'm not *entirely* anti-drone either. I do think that they have some valid and effective uses. If somebody gets caught in a riptide, and we're looking for a cheap, effective, and instantaneous means of searching for them, I think that a small fleet of drones could be a perfect solution.

Any type of technology can be used for evil though, and it's the use of drones for *sinister* purposes that I object to. That's what we saw throughout 2020. Drones were used as a surveillance agent extensively throughout the entire year to ensure that people were complying with the tyrannical and draconian unconstitutional public health regulations that they had passed.

We saw drones being used by police agencies throughout the world to enforce masking and social distancing while out in public. Many of these had facial recognition software. That way, not only would you have to worry about public shaming and being watched in public, but you would have to worry about potential government reprisal as well. Alabama State University actually purchased several of these types of drones so that they could spy on their students. After contracting with Dragonfly for "pandemic drones", ASU bought five Smart Thermal and Vital Sign Assessment Units, and five Social Distancing Awareness Units. The former drones actually have equipment with which they can monitor heart rate, respiratory rate, and oxygen saturation all within a few seconds of camera monitoring.[6]

We saw drones with thermal imaging technologies being used to monitor cityscapes to ensure that every last crevice of the city was complying with draconian "law". Chula Vista, California actually used night-vision capable drones to patrol the city at night to ensure that COVID regulations were being followed.[21] That is both a new level of surveillance, and a new level of invasion of privacy.

As with any new type of technology – with any new tool – we have to be incredibly careful that we're not dipping our toes into evil with how we use it. Potentially, a drone can be one of the greatest invaders of privacy that we have in the modern world. A drone is the potential to put a camera anywhere, anytime. It renders privacy fences, hedgerows, trees, walls, and any other form of privacy-creating barrier completely obsolete. All that's required to see what's on the other side is a drone and a smartphone. We now have full video and photographic access to whatever is happening on the other side.

Think about the implications of such. Let's say that for whatever reason, your wife enjoys topless sunbathing in your background pool. There's a substantial privacy fence built around your entire property, so you've never had to worry before about any peeping toms checking in on your wife. With the presence of drones, now you do. All a neighbor has to do is fly a drone directly above his own property high enough to see over your fence, and he can take all the pictures of your wife that he wants.

Where this becomes truly concerning is when this technology is used by the government. While the legal waters around this subject were murky at first, it appears now that it's been decided a homeowner does not own the airspace above his own home. The specifics of these types of laws will undoubtedly vary from location to location, but for the most part it's been decided that a homeowner only owns the airspace above their house that they could "reasonably use". As mentioned, what the reasonable amount of airspace that you own will be is going to vary depending upon where you live.

What this means though is that all a government-run drone has to do is fly a *foot* above the reasonable use threshold and they can collect all of the photos of your property that you want. This way they can avoid any pesky Bill of Rights restrictions on unwarranted searches of your privacy, and with a camera with adequate zoom, gather all the information about you that they want.

Are you running an apiary they now deem they have the "right" to inspect (an excuse to get on your property and snoop for something else)? Are you outside past curfew? Are you having a birthday party despite health code regulations? Are you reading political books that don't agree with the establishment on your back deck? Any of this can now be discovered in what they will deem to be a "legal" manner. They have used a loophole against you.

Now consider the fact that it would be incredibly easy to attach a listening device to these drones as well. Not only can video and images of your property be collected against your will, now they can listen to what you're saying as well. We've already established how governments across the globe have incorporated thermal imaging drones within their police and health departments. If such is flown over your neighborhood at night, will it be able to see who is having sex?

This is why we have to be *very* careful with the use of drones within the field of public health. They can very easily be turned from a useful tool (such as in search-and-rescue situations) to a tool for public surveillance and tyranny.

Artificial Intelligence (AI)

One of the most blatant and disturbing sources of privacy loss comes from artificial intelligence. When most hear the term "artificial intelligence" what instantly comes to mind is some autonomous and super-intelligent robot. This idea of a self-aware and sentient robot is actually referred to as "super-intelligence". Artificial intelligence is already all around us, it is simply that most people do not recognize it as such. The oft-quoted joke within the industry of robotics is that artificial intelligence is until it isn't. An AI software program is still AI, even once the mystery and magic are gone and the general public understand it.

For example, facial recognition technology often works off of AI software programs. Before we dive further into some of the consequences of such a technology though, let us first look at a few instances of how prevalent it is becoming, and what conclusions we may logically expect the future of AI to be drawn towards.

As of July 22, 2020, Artificial Intelligence Technology Solutions (AITS) stated in a press release that a major Hollywood studio had purchased two of the company's Robotic Observation Security Apparatus Units (ROSA for short). These had been purchased from AITS's subsidiary company Robotic Assistance Devices' dealer GSG Protective Services in LA, California.

This would ordinarily not be any big deal until you realize what it is that AITS has created. ROSA is an AI-driven security system that includes "both human and vehicle detection, license plate recognition, and complete integration with the RAD Software suite notification and response library." ROSA can also determine if you are wearing a mask or not, visually monitoring a 180-degree field of view. Facial recognition is used to identify those walking into the monitored perimeter, and those who refuse to wear a mask are recorded by ROSA, with individuals being tagged within the system if ROSA has identified them as repeat offenders of mask mandates.[19]

Here we see the very elements of what I am talking about. People have been made afraid of coronavirus, mask mandates have been created, and as a result we now have artificial intelligences beginning to roll out that police the public. Traffic cameras are regularly used to ticket individuals who they have deemed to have rolled a stop sign, run a red light, etc. It is not hard to foresee these types of AI's being used to send tickets to those who they find not socially distancing, not wearing a mask, engaging in an "illegal" gathering, or wearing clothing that is deemed to be hate speech. And to further add fuel to the fire, I personally know of a *church* that utilizes similar technology *within their foyer*.

When congregation members aren't wearing a mask, the AI recognizes such, announces via speaker that they need to wear a mask, and does who-knows-what-else with that congregation members biometrics. Does it use facial recognition to identify the church member? Does it keep track of repeat offenders? What is the church policy when it has identified repeat offenders of tyrannical laws? Does the pastor now turn over members of his flock to the police for punishment all because they prefer to breathe oxygen rather than carbon dioxide? Now, picture that. Why does a pastor, reverend, or bishop think that they have the right to monitor their congregation on such an extreme level whenever they are in the building? What do they do with such information? This should be a cause of hesitation for everyone.

And some technologies are better than others too. Don't forget that. The ACLU of Northern California found that facial recognition tech actually *misidentified* 26 members of the California legislature.[4] The ramifications of such a situation could be huge. Imagine being in court, accused of a crime which you did not commit. Perhaps you allegedly violated a lockdown order, weren't wearing a mask in public, or (gasp!) were found to have visited a Christmas party. You know for a fact that you did nothing but binge watch *The Mandalorian* all weekend at your house, but your arguments all seem to come to naught because the *AI* identified you at such-and-such a location. How well do you think your arguments will hold up in court? How much are you going to pay in court costs, hotel rooms, missed labor, and lawyer fees in order to clear your name?

Artificial intelligence – like drones – is a very powerful form of technology that we have to be very careful with if we don't want to unleash Frankenstein upon the public at large. Like drones, I can see where it could have its uses, but it will always place a massive amount of power into the hands of a select few individuals. We're talking about a level of power that will give a politician the capability to enforce just about whatever decree that he wants. Power corrupts and the amount of temptation that it places into the hands of men is often too great to be resisted. This is the reason that the United States was founded with a very explicit set of documents inhibiting the amount of power that could be granted to any one man, or any group of men. It is worth considering if we should think about how much power we are granting public health and police departments through the unlimited use of such technologies.

Contact Tracing

I understand the point of contact tracing. I received my master's in public health. I took those courses. Yet once more, there is a drastic difference between truly focusing on contact tracing and prying into peoples' private lives and even *tracking* them as they go about their daily business. Throughout 2020 we saw a number of public health department created apps that were designed "to assist in your safety". The argument ran along the lines of, "You want to keep safe, don't you? That's why you need our app."

Unfortunately for them, Amnesty International, a human rights group, performed a study on COVID-19 contact tracing apps and found that there were some rather dangerous security flaws in many of them. Apps for Norway, Bahrain, and Kuwait were found to actually transmit one's *real-time GPS data* and matched that data with one's personal identity. In essence, these apps were broadcasting your real-time location to whoever decided that they wanted to observe. What could be the possibilities here? Could this not make it ever easier for alphabet organizations to know when they can safely snoop through your belongings, papers, and files at home? If somebody higher up wanted to know when they could safely put a hit, would this not assist them? If they took a liking to your daughter, would this not help them determine when they could find her alone?

Despite these publicly revealed security flaws, nations such as Bahrain have credited their apps with being part of the reason that as of June 2020 that their death rate due to covid was 0.24%. It appears that the ends justifies the means, according to these people. It's perfectly acceptable to create a Big Brother society as long as it keeps people *safe*, right? The ironic thing about this is that a world where Big

Brother is always watching is anything but safe. Don't believe me? Read the history of Nazi Germany, Soviet Russia, China, or just about any other socialist/communist nation out there. It all ends the same.

These apps quickly turn into a form of policing as well. The way that they are created to work is to notify you when you come into contact with somebody who has been *diagnosed* positive for coronavirus. The apps send you a text when such has occurred, and then directs you to stay at home in quarantine for two weeks. If you refuse to do so, the government then knows because your phone will be set to notify the police should you leave a certain perimeter from your home. Your first thought when discovering this information is that you'll just leave your phone at home then. Unfortunately, that won't work either. The governments have already thought of this. You need those COVID apps in many cases to access businesses such as grocery stores.[22]

This is not just something that only happens in foreign countries either. "It couldn't happen here" is not a valid argument. Even the US is on board with much of this, depending on where you are located. A top Google executive stated via blog post on July 31, 2020, that Google had been in contact with 20 US states and territories (covering around 45% of the US population) to explore Google's new contact tracing programs.[23]

Further proving this point, it was in early August of 2020 that the Department of Homeland Security had documents released revealing that a private task force (called the COVID-19 Tech Task Force) composed of Big Tech companies (AWS, Camber, ESRI, Facebook, Google, Microsoft, Mozilla, R4, SAP, and Salesforce) had expressed interest in the *surveillance* capacity of covid tracking apps.

These apps typically utilize Bluetooth to determine if you have recently been in close proximity to anyone who has tested positive.[24] So yes, using contact tracing as a form of surveillance is already happening here within the US.

Private companies throughout the States have even resorted to making these types of apps *mandatory* for their employees. To begin with, this seems to be an encroachment by an employer on one's private property. If I pay for the phone and its memory, what right have *you* to *force* me to give you some of that data space? If it is a company phone, that is slightly different, but an employer does not have the right to an employee's personal property. It would be akin to an employer forcing you to let them utilize your home for business conferences or to use your car for making deliveries. Either option is theft and extortion. It's using the threat of taking away somebody's financial stability if they don't do something with their own private property you want them to do.

However, such a mindset – that extortion is ok – is rampant throughout America. As of August 14, 2020, there were a little over 50 new apps designed to "combat the spread of COVID-19". Employers across the country began to mandate their employees have one of these apps installed on their phones, or risk losing their ability to work, and therefore pay their bills. Public Citizen - a nonprofit consumer advocacy organization founded in 1971 - released a report that found around 340,000 workers were being monitored throughout the States by 32 different employers, and that nearly an additional 4 million workers were at risk of being surveilled should their 14,000 other employers actually activate the apps.

Aside from a change in the employee-employer contract that was written up when those employees began working those jobs, this is also an incredible cyber security risk. History has shown us that anybody can be hacked. Many businesses across the country actually fight dozens of hack attacks each day, and those companies must be successful in every single one, every single day. A hacker only has to win once. Once a hacker wins in retrieving that data, he now has a treasure trove of information, including personal health data, and (if contact tracing apps are being used) potentially even the GPS data of each employee that works for the hacked company.

We're going to assume that the hacker is a bad person. They just stole information, so this isn't a difficult conclusion to come to. There's a reason that corporate espionage is illegal. With his treasure trove of information, this hacker will likely have the "mug shot" of every employee hired by the company. Most large companies have a photo ID badge of some sort, so now this hacker will know what everybody looks like. He can now easily comb through the pictures to see if there are any images of women, he finds particularly attractive. If he now has their GPS data as well, you can imagine what some of the end results could be.

And all for what? For the illusion of safety.

Burcu Kilic, the digital rights program director for Public Citizen points out the futility of it all when he states, "None of them [the apps] have been proven to be effective at mitigating the spread of COVID-19."[25] If we know that these apps don't work, why are they being mandated? Perhaps there is a more sinister purpose at play? I'll leave you to ponder over that one on your own.

And this mandating of contact tracing apps doesn't even cover the fact that we are now encouraging, enabling, and allowing employers *to invade their employees' private health information*. Both Microsoft and UnitedHealth's

ProtectWell app send COVID diagnostic test results directly to the employer, bypassing the patient.

Since when does an employer have the right to instantly receive an individual's medical test results on anything? What should happen if the employee would much rather not have the entire company know that he tested positive? Why can't he quietly request from his boss that he take two weeks off of sick time? Where does this end? Will we begin sending STD diagnostic test results directly to the employer? What are the statistics of co-workers who end up in relationships with one another? Could that not be a problem with worker safety? What happens if science determines that certain sexual practices are associated with COVID-19? Does this not then help to stigmatize the patient? Ask anyone who has tested positive for coronavirus, and they will likely attest feeling like they were treated as a leper when around their friends and coworkers. They were treated *differently* after people had discovered that they had a certain type of infection.

This is why HIPAA was put into place. It was to protect an individual's privacy. Reputations and lives can be ruined when information gets out into the public world that the public world never had a right to in the first place. People can very easily end up being discriminated against.

The same would likely happen should your entire workplace be told that you suffered from anal leakage, chronic halitosis (bad breath), or went to the ER last year with a Barbie doll shoved up your rectum. All of these have actually happened – as a healthcare professional, I can tell you that all of them are constant diagnoses. This is the reason that medical information is inherently understood to be *private* information within HIPAA. Our current contact tracing efforts severely undermine any form of privacy at the foundational level.

College students are not immune to these types of infringements on their privacy either. During 2020 some colleges throughout the US required that their students install contact tracing apps on their phones, further turning their smartphones into tracking devices for even more eyes to browse.[6] Does a college president need to know where your 19-year-old daughter is at all times? Is such information truly of use to him? Is it truly necessary to collect?

Reports from other universities include students having to swipe their student ID every time they enter a new building, floor, or room. The thinking behind such is that this will help assist with contact tracing efforts. I've personally spoken with a student from such a school. They informed me that they receive multiple alerts via their phone *per day* telling them that they were just recently exposed to a positive COVID case just a day or so before. At this point, how is this assisting anybody? When somebody is being notified every day, what are they supposed to do, just sit on their bed all day? It's the story of the boy crying wolf on steroids. The fact of the matter is that these types of apps and notification systems truly do not work. Unless, of course, you are using them to track your *students* rather than a virus. In that case, they work like a charm.

Even your crap is not safe from being inspected and monitored. Researchers throughout the US have been tracking the course of COVID cases by monitoring sewage as it flows into government-owned channels. Summit County, Utah stated that they saw a decline in coronavirus presence within sewage after new anti-virus measures were incorporated. Not too far away in Cache County, Utah, it was found that sewage had revealed an outbreak of COVID at a meatpacking plant days before it was officially reported.[26]

How would you feel if you discovered that government agents were digging through every trash bag that you left out by your mailbox, taking pictures of their findings? Though such an action is most certainly not illegal – you did throw that trash out, after all – would such not be disturbing? And what are the consequences if the government decides that you didn't take appropriate action soon enough? You may have been asymptomatic for two days – maybe even had a slightly runny nose – but your poop decreed that you had COVID two whole days before you actually began to self-quarantine. Could such information then be used in a court of law to find you liable for other cases that happened as a result of you? If COVID could be used in a court of law as such, why couldn't flu, chickenpox, mono, or STDs? And if the government can monitor your sewage, is it too far of a step to think that they could easily decide to fine you if you had COVID positive sewage, but didn't self-quarantine in time?

The fining and imprisonment of those who have fought against quarantine and contact tracing has already happened. New York Commissioner of Health, Dr. Patricia Schnabel Ruppert, threatened those who didn't comply with her contact tracing efforts with both subpoenas and $2000 per day fines.[27]

So, if you went to your grandfather's birthday party - which you had kept private information because you didn't feel that the entire world needed to know - somebody later tested positive for COVID, and then contact tracers showed up to your home and you promptly told them to screw themselves and go home (not wanting to turn your grandfather in to the authorities), you could then face a court date. *All for spending time with your family.* This is a level of power that nobody in American office of any sort holds.

Michigan's governor - Gretchen Whitmer - attempted to do the same, deciding that she has the "right" to know who is going out to eat and when. As of the week of November 2, 2020, Michigan diners were required by Whitmer to give their full name and contact information to restaurant staff any time that they went out to eat. All in an attempt to assist with contact tracing. Those who violate the executive order could be fined $1000, given a misdemeanor, and even potentially face imprisonment. All for not telling the restaurant who you are and your phone number. If the restaurant staff doesn't comply with the executive order, they could end up causing their employer to have his business license revoked, and thus, be out of a job.[28]

I imagine there were some who sidestepped this order via the use of a masked phone number from MySudo.com, a Mission Darkness faraday cage around their phone to keep their cell phone from being pinged (tracked), a fake address, and a fake name. I further imagine there were diners in Michigan who used Reflectacles anti-facial recognition glasses throughout this time as well so that they couldn't be identified by such technology.

But I digress. The point is that contact tracing is to be used to truly assist in containing infectious disease. It's not to be used to track a populace, to serve tyranny, or as a qualifying factor for holding a job. Like drones, like AI, contact tracing can be a powerful tool, which is why it must be used by those who fully understand the risks to freedom that it poses and what can be done when it is weaponized by those with nefarious purposes.

Creation of The Snitch Force

Though Orwell's Big Brother idea of cameras being ever-present was most certainly a forewarning of what was to come, the fact of the matter is that cameras simply cannot catch *everything*. There are always going to be some "dark zones" that they will inevitably miss. If you truly want to ensure that every jot and tittle of whatever your political mandate is will be followed to a tee, then you have to break through the last barrier that is keeping you from reaching your goals: human trust.

This is accomplished by getting your constituents to do your spying and surveilling *for* you. Every totalitarian government of modern history has put such a policy into use. Whether it be Mao's China (shoot, even current China), Stalin's Russia (or again, current Russia), Nazi Germany, Fascist Italy, or a wide number of other options, people lived in fear of one another because people snitched on one another. Any government that advocates for such – advocates for friends and families turning against each other for truly unreasonable crimes – is arguing for the growth of totalitarianism, and this should be readily recognized as such and resisted.

It is a common factor of the totalitarian state to turn the people against one another. In such an environment, the government needs to ensure that the populace as a whole will comply with its every whim and fancy, and the best way to do this is to instill fear in its populace. Heavy fines and other forms of stiff punishments most certainly need to be used in order for this to happen, but they are often not enough. No matter how many cameras, trackers, microphones, and so on that the government utilizes, the fact remains that they cannot be everywhere all at once.

There will still be plenty of illegal activity taking place that goes against the government's wishes, and this not only undermines the totalitarian state's end goals, but it undermines the level of authority and power that the people at large deem the state to have as well.

If people do not view the state as truly being all-powerful, then they will in turn ignore the state's decrees, and this is very dangerous and embarrassing to those who are making such decrees. As a result, one of the most effective ways that the state can ensure that its directives are being obeyed to the letter and without fail is to create a snitch force. If you can ensure that people cannot trust their own friends, neighbors, relatives, parents, spouses, and *even children*, then you can better ensure that they will follow whatever directive you give them.

For example, when we hear that as of November 2020, children in Vermont are going to be questioned by school authorities after the Thanksgiving break to determine if their parents properly followed coronavirus restrictions, can we truly say that this is anything other than totalitarianism? Such actually happened!

Governor Phil Scott – a man who has the audacity to call himself a Republican (when in fact he's a Collectivist) – issued an executive order that prohibited gatherings of any kind between households. It didn't matter if your Thanksgiving party was going to be inside or outside, socially distanced or not, Phil Scott decreed that you could not celebrate Thanksgiving, and it must be so. The Vermont Agency of Education then directed schools to ask students if they were part of multi-family gatherings for Thanksgiving. If the answer was yes, then those students were required to engage in distance learning – where the student has to attend classes online – for 14 days. If the students couldn't do that, then they were told they must utilize distance learning for 7 days then get tested for COVID, stated Scott.

This mandate was justified by Vermont Education Secretary Dan French by his saying, "Schools operate on trust with their parents and their students, and we're hopeful this guidance will give them some additional tools to help everyone do the *right thing* and keep school safe. [emphasis added]" So not only do we have the state encouraging *children* to turn in their *parents*, but we have them saying that *this is the right thing*. The argument is raised that doing such will keep the schools safe. Yet does anyone see how this could be very dangerous to the personal liberty of those families affected by such an executive order?

It's interesting to note as well that Scott's executive order made exceptions for workplaces and retail stores.[29] In other words, it was *perfectly* safe to go to Food Lion, Walmart, Lowe's, or your cubicle farm, but for goodness' sake, don't have Thanksgiving dinner with your family. That is *dangerous*. Perhaps families could have worked around the order by celebrating Thanksgiving together at Walmart? Would that have been a safe alternative?

Such executive orders raise the question if whether or not they are truly about stopping a supposed pandemic, or whether they are *actually* about something else. It seems to me that when a decree is made with such apparent logical holes within it, that an incredibly degree of suspicion must be raised. It brings support to fears that there is a deeper agenda at play.

One of the earliest examples of the creation of a snitch force within the United States came from New York's Bill de Blasio in April of 2020, when he encouraged residents to turn in anybody that was found not following COVID regulations. This came in the form of a tweet saying, "How do you report places that aren't social distancing? It's simple: just snap a photo and text it to 311-692." Ironically, de Blasio was caught on film on April 17, 2020, without a mask while addressing a crowd of people in a hospital.[30]

This idea of a snitch force continued to infect other state governments, moving on to the islands of Hawaii. It was there in June 2020 that former reporter Angela Keen created a Facebook group called the Hawaii Quarantine Kapu Breakers ('kapu' means rules, in Hawaiian) where members could spy on vacationers' social media pages, looking for COVID violations within these images, which would then promptly be turned over to police.

Angela's group of Stasi agents had led up to 35 arrests of vacationers by June 25, 2020. It was due to the public providing this information themselves that a legal loophole was provided that kept police from being sued. Lt. Audra Sellers, a Maui police spokesman had this to say, "As a small community here in Hawaii, it takes everybody to be able to keep everybody safe...You know, some people say, 'Oh, you're snitching on people,' but that's not how you see it. It's seen as the fact that you want to keep the community safe."[31]

Well, if all that's necessary to justify a government overreach is to say, "Well, that's not how I see it..." then how can one be wrong? Can we not then justify anything? All we then have to do is have a different opinion!

Hawaii and New York weren't the only states with snitch lines though. Cuyahoga County in Ohio had also created a hotline residents could call if they caught others not abiding by COVID regulations. The number (216.698.5050) could be called by anyone, and county workers would then be put into contact with the complained about party to let them know that a complaint had been filed against them. From there, the complaint would be forwarded to the Board of

Health and the relevant city or village. If the hotline received repeated complaints about any particular American citizen, the sheriff's department would then be notified and sent out to both investigate and potentially file charges.[32]

Virginia's Governor Northam fell into a similar camp with the creation of a government snitch force website in which one could turn in suspected violations of COVID regulations to the government. Amongst this list of locations subject to stringent COVID regulations/lockdowns were gun ranges and churches – a blatant violation of both the First and Second Amendment. And to make matters even worse, all of these complaints could be made anonymously![33] Businesses could then snitch on their competitors, ex-girlfriends could snitch on their former boyfriends, and Common Core/Critical Race Theory-teaching public schools could then snitch on Christian private schools. As you can see, the potential for serious victimization of citizens is very large here.

Even private companies weren't immune to the temptation to play their turn at being Big Brother. Uber jumped on the bandwagon as well in July 2020, when they stated that they would begin participating with local health authorities to help with contact tracing for free. Uber made it so that every time you utilized their services, Uber could track you to see if you've been in contact with any COVID-positive people. If a prior rider in the cab was found to be COVID-positive, Uber would then send *your* personal information to a health authority as well. This all came about with Uber's policy stating that it both can and will disclose user information to public health agencies during an emergency.[34]

As expected, the idea of a snitch force flourished in other nations as well. It was in September of 2020 that the

Policing Minister of the UK, Kit Malthouse, suggested that people should spy on their own friends and families and report them if they were caught violating COVID regulations. This came about after England's "rule of six" mandate was passed, making groupings of more than six people illegal if those people were not all of the same household. Violation of this mandate resulted in a fine of between 100-3200 pounds, and anyone hosting a house party was liable to a 10,000 pound fine.

Simultaneously, the British government announced that they were creating "Coronavirus Marshals" – a new police force agency – to go about patrolling towns and cities enforcing social distancing, amongst other COVID regulations.[35] For a country that had previously spent time fighting against such government overreach (World War II), this is an excellent example of humanity's tendency to fall into forgetfulness.

Oregonian Governor Kate Brown seemed to like the British "rule of six" though for she ended up creating a similar mandate in her own state. She banned groups of more than six in private homes just days before Thanksgiving, telling her constituents to report others to police who were found violating this COVID edict. Brown said, "This is no different than what happens if there's a party down the street and it's keeping everyone awake. What do neighbors do? They call law enforcement because it's too noisy. This is just like that. It's like a violation of a noise ordinance."[36]

How a family getting together to see each other once more for a holiday is comparable in any way shape or form to keeping an entire community awake at 2AM is beyond me, but things did not have to make sense in 2020. They just seemed to happen regardless of what the supreme law of the land – The Constitution – said. Politicians and health officials truly just did whatever they felt like.

But what is the crux of the matter? What is the end point that we are trying to make? It's this: encouraging citizens to snitch against one another for a politician's fancy – encouraging families to turn against one another in service of the state – is morally reprehensible. Such has no place within the realm of public health whatsoever, and to encourage such so that public health regulations will be followed is to breach human rights.

3

Numbers

"The liberties of a people never were, nor ever will be, secure, when the transactions of their rulers may be concealed from them." – Patrick Henry

It was Plato who argued that those within the governing politik of people have the right and duty to tell "noble lies" to get people to do what the authorities wanted them to do. This is utter nonsense, and a rather Machiavellian view of life. It is nothing short of manipulation.

Though there are certainly instances (such as war) where there is going to be information that needs to be kept secret from the public at large, overall, government should be as transparent and truthful as possible. Particularly within the span of public health, we need to know that what we are being fed is not an outright lie. How can any man decide what is best for his own self and his family should the information he is being constantly fed by the government nothing such?

I am most certainly not arguing for one's unwavering trust in government offices. To argue for such – or even to believe in it – would be a new level of naivety and stupidity. But there should be truth behind something as basic as disease information. If there is an epidemic or local outbreak of some kind – whether that be an STD, flu, or vaping-related health problem - that the public does need to know about, then the public should have access to actual reliable data so that they can make the best decision for themselves (not having the government making such a decision for them). This can easily be done without violating individual privacy by not attaching personal information to case data.

But what is to be said when the numbers appear to be being made up? What is to be said when the numbers are willingly being handled carelessly despite a knowledge that public policy is being created from them? Did this happen throughout the United States in 2020? Let us take a look.

It was in a May 11, 2020 New York Times piece that we were told that a third of all US COVID deaths were found to be in either nursing home residents or nursing home workers.[1] It wasn't but 15 days later that the CDC admitted that it was possible that "less than half of those testing positive will truly have antibodies", thus saying that less than half of the positive antibody tests could be correct.[2]

A 50% margin of error is rather drastic, wouldn't you say? Around the end of June of 2020, the CDC announced that about 25 million Americans *may* have contracted COVID. Let us come back later to the efficacy of announcing to a people how many of them *may* be sick. The figure of 25 million was 10x higher than the actual number of confirmed cases (2,407,167 as of June 25, 2020). Robert Redfield, the CDC director, said that the reason that this many cases may exist is due to many of these people having been asymptomatic.[3]

So if we're going to admit that roughly 25 million people *may* have coronavirus, yet they were asymptomatic, aren't we building mountains out of molehills? Do we really have a problem if we have a disease that doesn't even cause symptoms in the majority of people who test positive for it?

Later, in July, the Texas Department of State Health Services removed 3484 cases from the total Texan COVID count because the San Antonio Metro Health District was found to be including *probable* cases in their case totals. The reason this was happening was that in Texas, people can be considered a positive COVID case even if they haven't gotten a PCR test. All they have to do to be considered positive is to meet two of the three following criteria: possessing COVID-like symptoms, close contact with a positive COVID case, and getting a positive antigen test.

This means that within Texas, if you go to the doctor with a cough and have been in contact with a positive case, you are considered an official COVID positive case in the official statistics.[4] This is an incredibly easy way to pad the numbers. As we've already discussed within the chapter on contact tracing, it is very easy to make it appear as if the entire nation has had direct exposure to a "positive" on a daily basis. With contact with a positive case being a qualifier, this makes it so that anybody in Texas with the flu, a cold, allergies, or any other health condition that could cause something as minor as just a sore throat or a runny nose could easily be classed as a positive case.

Stringent and respectable testing criteria must always be the norm when it comes to a reportable disease. Numbers are used to craft health policy, and they need to be realistic. Furthermore, something could easily be said for the fearmongering that comes from leading the public to believe that the greater portion of the nation is infected with a life-robbing illness, and that there are likely "asymptomatic" around you on a daily basis spreading the disease throughout communities. The only thing that this does is to create panic and stir up hatred, vitriol, and ultimately, violence against one's own neighbors, friends, and countrymen.

Problematic Testing

One of the chief problems with COVID testing was the length of time that it took to receive back test results. At least within my own community, it was not uncommon to *not* receive results for at least a week. I even heard of cases in my town that took roughly 14 days to get test results back from. How is it that we can get flu test results back in about 10 minutes, but we have to wait days in order to get COVID tests back?

If we *truly* are concerned that there is an infectious disease running rampant throughout our communities, doesn't it make sense that we get our test results back as quickly as possible? If we *truly* do have an infectious disease crisis on our hands, this is the only ethical option. To wait for any unreasonable amount of time otherwise is to condemn others to a similar fate. As the tested patient spends a week going about their business, shopping, working, working out, and the like, only to receive their positive test results back two weeks later, have we really done anything beneficial, or was our hesitation nothing more than a reason that the disease was spreading so rapidly?

I understand systems growing to be overloaded, but the reports that I am personally familiar with when COVID tests were taking a week plus to get back were from February – May, when we truly didn't have a lot of diagnoses. It was mismanagement (or worse) to the extreme.

Within *any* epidemic, prompt test results are the only ethical choice that we have. Time is essential at this point, and there could be dire consequences if we do not stress this. Imagine being forced to wait a week to be told that, yes, you were indeed having a heart attack after all. Imagine waiting 8 days to be told that yes, you did have appendicitis. That, yes, it *was* a stroke.

There would be public outrage, and rightfully so! So, *why*, if we truly believe that this is an incredibly contagious and incredibly dangerous virus – so much so, that it deserves the largest quarantine in history and the world's first *global* economic shutdown – are we waiting longer to receive test results than we did with Africa's Ebola crisis? Why are we waiting longer to get results from this supervillain of a bug than we are for your average flu test? It just doesn't make sense, does it?

The next problem with testing for infectious diseases or medical conditions, is that we need to ensure that whatever test we are using, that it has a high degree of accuracy and reliability. Throughout 2020, the means of testing for COVID were primarily what are called PCR tests. Unfortunately, PCR tests generate a *huge* number of false positives. Don't believe me? Just look to Africa, where even a mango was tested for COVID and was found to be a positive case.[5] The problem is the sensitivity of the PCR tests that we used throughout 2020. They were created *so* sensitive that people were testing positive for coronavirus infections that they had had years prior to 2020. Even genetic fragments of old virus bodies could trigger one to have a positive COVID test using the PCR testing criteria.

The presence of viral particles picked up by such a technique does *not* link to an active symptomatic infection. There simply doesn't appear to be any correlation there. Instead, it is the *cycle threshold* of a test that is a more important indicator of disease. If somebody has a low cycle threshold (CT) count, then that means that individual is absolutely loaded with the virus. They are probably someone that is currently contagious – if it is a contagious illness that is being tested for. In contrast, a high CT value means that there is a low viral load.[6]

Those are the figures that we should be looking at for testing, but they are most certainly not the ones that we are utilizing.

This was regularly pointed out as well. Dr. Michael Mina, an epidemiologist at the Harvard T.H. Chan School of Public Health agreed that the current testing procedures were much too sensitive. Why? Because a PCR test only searches for genetic material being present. It does not tell you how much genetic material is present. What does this mean in practice? People with insignificant amounts of genetic markers will be diagnosed as positive. As The Blaze reported in August of 2020, "Up to 90% of individuals who have tested positive for COVID-19 potentially carried such 'insignificant' amounts of the virus that they were not contagious." The New York Times said that roughly 6 million of the US COVID cases were thus likely not contagious.[7]

It was because of these faulty PCR tests that the University of Arizona had to issue an apology to student athletes there who the University told were positive for COVID. Initially, the university told 13 students that they had tested positive. After reanalyzing, it turned out that only two were actually positive.[8]

Better safe than accurate or effective, I suppose.

Why could such a form of testing even prove to be dangerous? Because there are always wicked and ignorant men who are going to be present in government that will look for any excuse they can to infringe on the unalienable rights of a people. For example, of such, just look at July 2020's Brooks County, Texas. It was there that those who were diagnosed as a positive COVID case were told that if they were caught out in public after receiving a positive test that they would be subjected to Texas Penal Code 22.05(1), which states, "A person commits an offense if he recklessly engaged in conduct that places another in imminent danger of serious bodily injury."

This was used to threaten jail time to those who would not comply with quarantine. David T Garcia, the Brooks County Attorney signed the notice stating that such would take place, saying, "Appearing in public after testing positive except to get medical care, can lead to your arrest."[9]

Do you see how such an inaccurate form of testing could easily prove dangerous? Imagine having seasonal allergies and going to your doctor to see if there's not some type of medicine you can get to counter the symptoms. The doctor decides it's a good idea to do a COVID test – he's been doing them on every patient that comes in his doors (not uncommon) – and sticks a Q-tip up your nose. He comes back later to notify you that it's COVID that's causing your symptoms after all. You've had seasonal allergies for years, so you're fairly positive the doctor is wrong, but now you've subjected yourself to being placed under house arrest for the immediate future. If you go out to buy groceries, go to church, or anything else now with your seasonal allergies, you risk potential incarceration.

And what is to be done when people are told they are positive when in fact they've never even been tested? Tricare, a health care program of the US DOD Military Health System, told around 600,000 people that they were a positive case of COVID-19. Those notified were then asked to consider donating their blood for research. However, many of these people had actually *never been tested for COVID*. Humana later apologized for the error, saying that they had sent out the email by accident.[10]

Now keep in mind that in both of these cases we have large amounts of people falsely being told that they had a contagious illness. And not just any illness. This was an illness that virtually all of the mainstream media had convinced the world would lead to their dying a lonely death while attached to a ventilator. This problematic testing directly led to multitudes of people being subjected to an extreme level of mental distress, and for what? Imagine giving out false positives for cancer tests willy-nilly. Imagine the public outcry and potential legal problems that would arise from somebody's telling 600,000 people that they had a terminal illness such as mesothelioma. None of those 600,000 actually *did* have mesothelioma, but doctors were diagnosing people with such regardless.

It would be a legal nightmare, would it not? While false positives are most certainly a part of life – it's hard to create a test that is 100% accurate 100% of the time – to have this high or a rate of error is simply unacceptable. The end result is fear, anxiety, improper choices, and in some instances – despair.

Mismanaging the Data

If data is to be used to determine public policy, then the public deserves to have the data be as accurate and truthful as possible. When statistics are toyed with however, then a false narrative can be developed.

As of November 27, 2020, there had been roughly 262,000 official COVID deaths nationwide, with a mortality rate of roughly 2.1%. The majority of deaths listed were among those who were 65 or older. It was then though that Dr. Genevieve Briand of John Hopkins University published a study noting some critical accounting errors all the way up to the national level. The study noted that there is an average number of deaths every year throughout the US from a variety of factors (e.g. heart attack, stroke, drowning, etc.), and that these averages remain rather constant. Thus, for COVID to be of serious alarm, there would need to be a statistically significant increase in the average number of deaths within the US. The results of Briand's study, however, found that in actuality, *there was no significant change in the number of deaths throughout the US,* and that the 2019-2020 timeframe showed deaths that mirrored past trends in seasonal illnesses.

What this means is that COVID had had relatively *no* effect on deaths throughout the US. What *was* a concerning discovery though was that the spike in *diagnosed* COVID deaths correlated with a proportional decrease in the number of deaths due to other diseases and causes. The conclusion of this is that people who actually died from other causes (e.g. stroke, heart attack, cancer) were being labeled as COVID deaths. Pneumonia, influenza, respiratory diseases, and other factors are all incredibly likely to have been the true causes of death in many of these cases, yet COVID was given as the actual reason of death. In short, deaths were being misclassified.

This lines up with what the CDC actually admitted earlier in the year (2020) when they stated that 94% of COVID deaths occur with comorbidities. Furthermore, COVID death stats mirror the normal distribution for death amongst age groups, giving even further credence to the idea of COVID deaths being a recategorization of other causes. The end conclusion of this study was that COVID is not the killer disease that it is widely touted to be throughout the mainstream media. Briand's study was quickly removed from internet search engines.[11]

There are numerous problems with such happening, but perhaps the greatest is the way in which policy was impacted. Let us examine how mismanagement of healthcare data leads to poor public health policy next.

Using Numbers to Help Determine Policy

Any public health policy that is to be created should most certainly utilize statistics so that informed decisions can be made. For example, if it is discovered that those who utilize a particular chemical in their manufacturing process will create a gas cloud that travels up to 25 miles away and causes facial paralysis in 87% of those who it comes into contact with, something obviously needs to be done. In such a case, statistics has been used properly to create policy.

If it's discovered that 90% of those within a town of 200,000 people are infected with a pandemic form of Congo hemorrhagic fever, then there are a number of policy decisions that we can make from such data to help protect the public health of the rest of a nation/the surrounding locales.

However, it is absolutely vital that we are 100% confident in the statistics that we are receiving if we are to make good public health policy. While this is not to say that we are searching for guarantees – they do not exist within the world of applied statistics – it is to say that we need to incorporate models with a high degree of accuracy and reliability. If there is any reason to believe whatsoever that the statistics we are using in the creation of health policy have been tampered with – or are unreliable – then as policy makers we *cannot* use such statistics to craft policy in good conscience. To do so is to force a tyrannical decree upon a citizenry with no reasoning other than that it fits the whim of those in office and with the *alleged* power to do such.

At no point along the process should a public health officer craft a number out of their head – or purposefully mislead others – with statistics that they believe will further their agenda. Case in point for such occurred in December of 2020. It was then that Dr. Fauci admitted within a *New York Times* article that he hadn't given his true thoughts on how many people would need to be given a shot against COVID to result in herd immunity.

Why?

Because he was afraid the "truth" would discourage people from getting the shot. His initial response to the question had been somewhere between the range of 60-70%. In November 2020, he bumped that figure up to 70-75% of the population needing to take the COVID shot for herd immunity. The week prior to Christmas 2020, Fauci said between 75-80% of Americans would need to take the shot for herd immunity to result.

Then came the *Times* interview. It was here he upped his figure to approximately 90%. Why did he do this? According to Fauci, "When polls said only about half of all Americans would take a vaccine, I was saying herd immunity would take 70 to 75 percent. Then, when newer surveys said 60 percent or more would take it, I thought, 'I can nudge this up a bit,' so I went to 80,85."[12]

In other words, it was an ulterior motive – an agenda – that was causing Fauci to manifest numbers out of thin air. Doing so does not assist in keeping human rights in public health. Regardless of what a public health worker may believe, they need to keep the data as truthful as possible.

While it is always difficult to give somebody a percentage off the top of one's head regarding how successful a given medical treatment will be ("I'd say the surgery will have a 80% chance of success, Mr. Jones."), to purposefully change that number over time not because the science has changed, but because you believe that you can further push your agenda – whatever that may be – is to use numbers to determine policy that may/aren't truthful.

Numbers, statistics, epidemiology – all of these should be used to better inform a public health worker so that they can make a more informed public health decision. It must be remembered though that these are decisions that are going to impact the lives of others though, and as such, they are to be taken very seriously. To not do so is to risk abusing one's position.

Inflated Numbers

There shouldn't even be a need for a discussion to examine whether or not it is ethical to inflate numbers of *any* disease or condition in order to further an agenda, yet 2020 happened, and so an examination is required.

Let's say that you were responsible for the quarterly budget committee reports for your church. You have been placed in a position of trust and responsibility where it is anticipated you will be as truthful and as accurate as possible. However, something has happened within the church that you are not happy about. Perhaps you believe the church has grown too materialistic or even prideful, and that the only way the church will get back to "the right place" is by being humbled in some form of extravagant way. *You* believe the best way to steer the church in the direction *you* believe that it should be going is to pad the budget numbers so that it *looks* as if the church has more money than it actually does.

You think that by doing so you can help to get the church to make decisions that will ultimately result in your desired end outcome – for the church to go bankrupt. You believe that by going bankrupt, the church will be able to "right its heart" so that it will now "better rely on faith" than "to rely on mammon". It doesn't matter that – in truth – the church has *no* issue whatsoever with materialism, pride, or any lack of faith. All that matters is that such is *your* perception of the matter.

You know that nobody would ever listen to you if you were forthright with what you believe needs to happen to the church. They would never accept your message of selling all the furniture to provide money for charity which would force everybody to sit on the ground or stand throughout the entire service. But what's a little discomfort when it comes to providing for charity in such a way? Isn't another's need for food more important than a few hours of comfort? And so, you begin to regularly lie to the deacons, pastors, and elders within the church about where the church is at financially.

Sure enough, your plan begins to work. More and more missionaries are given monthly pledges of support as time goes on, two new full-time staff members are hired, and a new construction project is even planned. All as a result of your padding the numbers. Things are moving along smoothly, and you couldn't be more pleased with how things are turning out.

Within a year and a half, your deceit is realized, and the church has to file for bankruptcy. People lose their jobs, missionaries lose their financial support, a number of other local service opportunities are shuttered, and the bank ends up foreclosing on the property, leaving the church members (in a sense) homeless.

Everything that you had ever hoped for has been brought to fruition. There's even a huge rift created within the church that causes many of the members to split off amidst a host of angry words that will never be forgotten. Friendships have been permanently severed. Your name is dragged through the mud, but you consider this nothing more than religious persecution. You worked towards bringing the church to a state of humility, and your reputation is simply part of the cost. Yes, you lied on the budget reports, but the outcome was exactly what you had always hoped it would be.

In such a situation, would you be justified in your endeavors? Does the end justify the means? Don't forget that aside from outright lying with your accounting and presentations, you also violated a great deal of trust that had been placed in you. You've ruined lives, livelihoods, reputations, and service opportunities.

Any outsider examining such a situation would obviously point out the inherent flaws in believing such actions were justified. Yet how is it that public health workers – who did the *very same thing* – have been let off of the hook for such?

If you give somebody a positive incentive to perform some action, then they are likely to perform that action (should they deem the incentive to be large enough to warrant the effort/risk). Money is most certainly a positive incentive, and when trying to get somebody to engage in a particular behavior, it is often only a matter of asking, "How much?"

Throughout 2020, we witnessed fatal motorcycle accidents in Florida being labeled as COVID deaths, gunshot wounds to the head being labeled as such, as well as falling and dying from a hip fracture, dying from Parkinson's, and a number of other non-COVID related deaths as well.

I personally witnessed a half a dozen or so individuals come to me and say that their loved ones had been labeled as having died from COVID when they *knew* beyond a shadow of a doubt they had actually died from a heart attack, heart disease, or some other chronic condition they had struggled with for some time. When your wife watches you have a heart attack in the kitchen and die, I feel that she has a fairly good idea of what she's talking about.

Others throughout the US began to grow suspicious with some of these reports as well, and at least in Palm Beach County, the CBS12's I-Team looked into the matter. They examined the Medical Examiner's spreadsheet of people who had recently died of COVID within their county and found that 8 cases of COVID deaths didn't even have COVID listed as a contributing cause of death. In response to having this pointed out, the Medical Examiner's office stated that the 8 cases were actually errors.

Oopsy.

Within that same county, local resident Rachel Eade, brought a lawsuit against the local government for its mask mandates. She combed through the medical reports of her county and found that out of the 581 COVID listed deaths for her area, only 169 listed COVID without any contributing factors.[13]

Rachel's discovery seems to be right in line with what the CDC has admitted as well. They issued a report on August 28 of 2020 that stated that only 6% of COVID deaths listed the only cause of death to be COVID with no other comorbidities. The report states, "For deaths with conditions or causes in addition to COVID-19, on average, there were 2.6 additional conditions or causes per death." At the time of this report there had been 167,558 COVID deaths throughout the US. Utilizing the CDC frame of reference, this means that only 10,053 of those people died from COVID alone.[14]

Joan Hill, a 79-year-old South Carolinian grandmother, was one of these inflated statistics. Her family received notice that she had died due to "COVID-19 complications" on the death certificate. This, despite the fact that Joan had never even tested positive for the virus. Her family noted that she never even exhibited any of the signs or symptoms of COVID. What did she die from? Dementia – a disease that she had been struggling with for years.[15]

As the reader, you yourself have likely heard dozens of similar reports. Friends and acquaintances who died from completely natural causes, yet COVID was listed on the death report as the final cause of death.

So the question that must be asked then is this: Why?

Why on *earth* would padding the numbers be suggested in the first place. And nobody can in clear conscience deny the fact that numbers for COVID were padded all along. There are quite simply too many people who have definitive proof such has taken place to believe otherwise.

I personally believe that communism was at the root of such a decision. It is the only conclusion that makes any sense to me. It's the only conclusion that fits that hole in the puzzle of what was 2020. The growth of an all-powerful state and the push for America (and the world) to move more towards a communist utopia was the end game of a number of powerful entities throughout the world. By creating fear – and by using false, padded numbers to do so – policies could be "justified" that would pave the way for such a totalitarian nation.

While there are most certainly some out there who would disagree with me, I don't think that people would disagree with my saying that padding numbers of any type to further an agenda when one has been placed into a position of trust is nothing short of falsifying data. You are presenting a lie to people while portraying it as the truth. A transparent government is warranted by a people.

If you picture a group of 24 people who have been marooned on a deserted island, I believe that this point can be further made. The people soon realize that they need to elect a leader as there are too many heads trying to prod people in too many different directions. The 24 gather together for a vote, electing three men as the "head council". Any decisions that they make are final.

They've elected a head council of their own accord to better serve their own interests. In this way they can have a coordinated response to whatever it is that life throws their way next. Now imagine that the head council decides to keep access to the wrecked ship's radio solely for their own use. It's by constant monitoring of this radio that the head council realizes the search for survivors of the wreck has been called off. The head council doesn't want to eliminate hope, knowing that this is what's helping a lot of the survivors to hang on – the hope of rescue.

In such a case, would the head council – the peoples' government that they elected – have the right to not tell people the truth? Even more, would the head council have the right to lie to the people, telling them that search planes were canvassing the area night and day? Both cases would likely be answered with a 'no'. Why do we expect any different from a public health worker? Why is transparency seemingly avoided at all costs and justified with mental gymnastics when prior falsifications are pointed out?

Human rights only end up being at risk of violation when public health workers take such a stand. Whether the end result is people making overly risky decisions that they wouldn't have made otherwise – had the data been truthful – and end up dying/being maimed, or whether the end result is people living in a state of paralyzing fear due to the false belief that there is a pandemic erasing swaths of people from the globe, padding the numbers results in people making potentially harmful decisions. It must be avoided at all costs by all those who hold ethics in high regard.

4

School Closings

I'll begin with the statement that I am against any public school to begin with. I don't see why I am forced at the end of a gun to pay for somebody else's child's education. I fully understand the importance of education, but how can it be deemed justified to legally force somebody who doesn't want children to have to pay for those who do? On a more painful note, what about forcing those who *can't* have children to have to pay for those who can? Is this not adding insult to injury?

Within the field of public health there are times when epidemics and outbreaks will cause authorities to come to the conclusion that shutting down a school is the best idea. Lice, flu, norovirus, and more are all examples of reasons why schools have been shut down in the past. And I'm not entirely against such. If schools are truly spreading disease, then there does need to be something done.

2020 brought this topic to the forefront of a lot of peoples' minds. The fact of the matter is that people have become used to the system that the government has imposed on them. They *have* to send their children to school or else they face serious legal punishment. This has been ingrained in American society for decades now. As a result, parents have planned around the school system. Parents have figured out when their children need to be headed out the door to go to school, and when the parent needs to go to work, etc. Now what happens when the government throws a monkey wrench into the entire system (that it has created)? Should there then not be some form of grace permitted for those who have come to rely on a system and then have had it yanked out from under our feet?

Let's assume that there is a devastating pandemic sweeping the globe. It is incredibly contagious, mutates quickly, and kills the great majority of people who contract it. It is not picky in who it chooses. Both adults and children are susceptible to its ravages, and nobody is immune.

If such were indeed the case, I personally would have no problem with schools throughout the nation being closed. As it is now, parents are threatened with having social services called on them with the risk of government-sponsored kidnapping of their children if they do not send them to school. In such a situation, where school has been made mandatory for all at the risk of kidnapping and jail time, I believe that the only solutions to avoid pandemic exposure of children are for governments to either A) shut down their schools, or B) move to an alternate format.

However, within this hypothetical, there must be plenty of evidence and valid proof that whatever it is that is infecting people truly needs to be controlled. Schools have shut down due to influenza and norovirus outbreaks for decades, and there is no inherent moral failure in shutting down a school due to an outbreak of illness. Throughout 2020 this closure of schools reached unprecedented levels, however. In order to better understand how a public health worker can keep human rights in public health, it would be worth an investigation to see just how things have happened in the past. We learn from past failures and successes, and I believe I can prove that 2020 was filled with more of the former, particularly when it comes to forced school closures.

As mentioned above, plenty of scientific proof needs to be at hand in order to fully justify that schools should remain closed. This doesn't always have to be local proof either. If we live in an area that has been untouched by a pandemic, and we know that a short 45-minute drive away a reported 9% of school-age children have already died from the pandemic in the past week, it is most certainly worth considering thinking about our options. In 2020, the response was to take this extreme approach – of a hard shut down across the board – without such data though. So the question is – in such a case – in 2020 - was it really worth it? Was a proper decision made here? Let's examine the evidence.

As of July 16, of 2020, more kids had died from the flu rather than COVID. Unlike COVID, however, the flu deaths that *did* occur in children occurred in *healthy* children. Throughout the 2017-2018 flu season – which was considered a pandemic as well – there were roughly 600 kids throughout the US who were killed due to influenza. The CDC conducted a study in 2018 that found after analyzing six different flu seasons that half of all flu deaths were in otherwise healthy children, and that 22% of those deaths were among those who were fully vaccinated against influenza as well.

When kids end up contracting the flu, they often end up bedridden for a week or more with a high fever, coughing, and muscle ache. When kids test positive for COVID though, almost all of them are either asymptomatic or very mildly symptomatic. Even when it comes to community spread, children were shown to barely contribute to spreading

COVID. Such is *not* the case with flu, however. Kids do contribute to the spread of influenza substantially.

Thus, to be consistent, if the government is going to mandate kids wear masks all day when they are allowed to go to school, and attend virtual classes at home when they aren't allowed to go to school – and all due to COVID – shouldn't they do the exact same thing every year from November to April? That's when flu season is after all, and it has proven to be much more dangerous to kids than COVID – *and* there was a vaccine for flu at the time, while there *wasn't* one for COVID (during 2020).

We vaccinate our kids against flu and then send them to school, something most have no problem with. California discovered during its 2017-2018 flu season that of the 187 reported ICU and fatal cases of flu amongst kids, 50.8% of the kids had received their flu shot for that year.[1]

So, what's the point?

Despite these statistics, the mainstream media and public health officials constantly harped about the importance of keeping schools closed in order to protect the community at large. This resulted in distance learning becoming commonplace throughout the country by July 2020. Let us take a closer look though. Where school-age children really a threat to the community? A study in Germany sought to answer this question. It was at the medical faculty of the TU Dresden and University Hospital that Carl Gustav Caru, found that the transmission of COVID among younger people was rare. His researchers took 2045 blood samples from students and teachers across 13 secondary schools and found that *only 12* of the samples were found to contain COVID antibodies. It's important to note that all of these tests were carried out in schools where there had been known (diagnosed) COVID outbreaks. Even 24 of these participants had at least one confirmed COVID diagnosis in their home, and of those 24, only one study subject had COVID antibodies. Thus, the study found that schools do not become the viral hotspots that the media painted them to be once they reopen.[2]

Again though, nothing seemed to change, and the panic painted by the media only seemed to grow worse. This – in spite of – the facts. When New York reopened 1800 public schools, three weeks into the in-person school year, the data proved that there was a surprisingly small number of positive cases. New York performed 16,298 random tests (we'll avoid the ethical qualms of such for now) throughout their schools and found that only *20* staff members (0.12% of all the random tests performed) ended up testing positive. Throughout New York City, only *8* students tested positive for COVID, and there was zero evidence of serious illness amongst those 8 kids either.

Icelandic researchers took things a step further. They sequenced the genomes of *every single positive case* throughout their country and failed to find a *single instance* of a child infecting patients. And what about child-care centers? Shouldn't they then become viral hot spots as well? The media seemed to paint such as truth through repetition. *True* science proved otherwise though. A study published in the *Journal of the American Academy of Pediatrics* performed a survey of over 57,000 day cares throughout the US, finding no association whatsoever between exposure to child care and COVID diagnosis.

And yet what was the response of such? Well, in Fairfax County of Virginia, the teacher's union demanded that schools remain closed for the remainder of the school year (it was October at that time). This demand came at a time when there were only 6 student infections per 100,000 in

Virginia during the first two weeks of October.[3] That comes out to 0.006% being infected.

And such sentiments were common. With the Fairfax County teacher's union, it most likely wasn't fear, but greed that drove such sentiments. These were government employees who were already paid a full year's work for roughly 9 months of work, with Christmas, Easter, and fall breaks. Fear can be a convenient disguise for laziness. Such happenings were fueled by organizations such as the American Federation of Teachers. They provided legal, financial, and staffing support for local chapters that went on strike due to COVID. The AFT ended up actually saying that they would only support fully reopening schools (their jobsites) if the average daily community infection rate was below 5% and the transmission rate was below 1%.[4]

New York's teachers went even further. One of its teachers' unions announced in August that NYC teachers might not even show up if *every* student and staff member was not tested for COVID prior to entry for in-person teaching. The president of the United Federation of Teachers, Michael Mulgrew, said, "Every single person – both adult and child – that is to enter an New York City school must have evidence that they do not have the COVID virus."

Keep in mind that there are more than 1 million students that attend NYC schools, and that number doesn't even include faculty and staff. On a daily basis, NYC conducted anywhere between 50,000 – 80,000 tests, with people often having to wait up to two weeks (as of August 2020) before getting their test results back.[5]

Government employees were essentially holding a gun against the head of the medical system of New York by threatening to not educate children (who's education had been paid for by taxpayer dollars), but also by threatening to clog the healthcare system of their entire state – causing those who truly *needed* medical help to not be able to access it in a timely fashion – and threatening the individual freedom of all those who they worked to serve as well.

It must be nice to be a government employee. To get a full year's wages for a fraction of its duration and to still believe that you are entitled to walk over the freedom of the people who pay your salary.

Such behavior and "logic" was common for New York throughout 2020 though. It was in November that NYC Mayor Bill de Blasio threatened to shut down all public schools once more, saying parents need to have a contingency plan as a result. This came from a state with some of the strictest COVID regulations throughout the US, and yet still facing what was termed a "second wave" of COVID. So, what did they decide to do? The exact same thing that apparently worked so well for them with the "first wave".

De Blasio also said, "learning bridges programs, which provide free childcare for kids in grades 3k to the 8th grade" would remain open, as well as "children in pre-k and 3k programs run by community-based groups."[6] COVID must mysteriously not attack those locations. Can we just send people *there* instead to teach the kids?

To move back to the point that must be made though, what are we to do regarding public schools, and even our university systems if there is some type of dire pandemic type event? If we have an incredibly contagious illness (bacterial, viral, fungal, parasitical, or other) that is sweeping the nation, and which has the potential to make millions of people very sick or worse, then we *do* have to do something.

We cannot rightfully force people to send their children to school in such a situation. To do so is to expose them to a very real risk of illness or death, and to expose their families to the same. So what is to be done?

I believe that the solution to this dilemma is twofold. First, have an at-home contingency plan that can easily be implemented if need be, so that students can still continue to learn while in the safety of their own homes. This allows adjustments to be made in the school year with minimal interruptions. For example of such, let's say that there's been a norovirus outbreak at several school campuses within your county.

In such an instance, school administrators have consulted with health officials and found that the norovirus will die off of the surfaces that it's currently on within the school in 7-10 days. If the school decides that shutting down the physical premises for this amount of time is wise so that the remaining 2/3rds of the school doesn't end up sick, this decision can easily be implemented without the students missing a week's worth of school *if* there is an at-home contingency plan ready to be implemented at a moment's notice.

While nobody out there will argue the point that online learning is just as effective as in-person teaching, this type of system being put into place at least helps to ensure that there is some learning going on within the span of that week. However, I do believe that it is also unfair to assume that everybody out there has internet access.

Those who live in more rural environments very rarely have access to high-speed internet, if access to internet at all. It is unjust to force children to attend a public school and then also mandate that if they don't purchase some type of internet (which very well may be outside of their means) that they will fall behind in their education or be harmed on their report cards. Good grades on report cards *do* truly matter, and poor report cards can easily be the difference between a student receiving a necessary scholarship for a college. We need to ensure that we're not harming students' abilities to receive a good grade solely due to not having internet access at home. If a student earns a bad grade of their own accord, well, such is on them. That is a consequence of their own decisions.

However, if in a class full of 50 students, 3 of them receive a failing grade not because they are poor students but because they do not have internet access at home and after shifting to a solely online course format, they weren't able to complete assignments, then we do have an issue. If you are going to mandate online work, you are also mandating that the student's parents purchase computers, modems, routers, and an internet provider.

That is very important to remember.

If you're going to solve this problem by giving every student a tablet or laptop of some kind so that they can work on their homework at home, the student still may not have access to internet at home. If over a month's span that student hasn't turned in any assignments (they're 14, can't drive, live in a rural environment, and they come from a single-parent home where the mother works all day), it is not because the student hasn't wanted to be a good student, but instead because you have set the student up for failure with your policy. And yes, while I understand that virtually every person on the planet nowadays has had their life completely changed by Steve Job's creation of the smartphone, there will still be outliers.

And here's why we have to be careful with mandating alternative schooling formats:

While switching to online formats is potentially understandable, this government action created a host of other problems. Parents who had relied on schools for years as a form of "day care", if you will, suddenly had to figure out a way for their children to be watched throughout the workday until the parent got home. You can't exactly leave a 5 and an 8-year-old at home all day by themselves and expect things to still be in one piece when you get home from work. Likewise, parents who didn't have internet coverage at their residence, whether that be due to financial constraints, rural geography, or other reasons were left out in the dust. In the case of those who couldn't afford internet coverage, they now had another expense forced upon them by the government – *at risk of having their children kidnapped from them.* For those who did not have internet due to a rural location, they were systematically being punished for not living within an urban environment. Their parents' home choice/lifestyle was deemed as sufficient reason to punish the children with the threat of kidnapping.

And such did occur.

Parents throughout Massachusetts in August of 2020 told the newspaper *The Boston Globe* that they had been reported to the Department of Children and Families for neglect because their children had been absent too many times from the state's remote learning options. This happened immediately after the entire state of Massachusetts switched over to online formats for student learning. No grace period was given to learn the ways to work around the new system that the government had imposed on thousands of parents state-wide – they were simply reported to the authorities. The great majority of these parents reported were mothers, many of which had had no prior involvement with social services. Some of these mothers reported having reached out to the school system for assistance in balancing the situation – between work, being a parent, and teaching their children – and were not given any help. If those charges of neglect were upheld by the DCF, those parents could risk having their children taken away from them.[7]

This is wickedness to the extreme. It is a violation of human rights on a number of different levels. Aside from the forcing of a student to attend a public school, there is also the forcing of a parent to pay for an internet provider, a computer, a router, a modem, and all of the other necessary accoutrements of rural online access. It's to set a child up for failure, and then threaten to take him from his family and throw him in a foster care home where the threat of mistreatment, sexual abuse, or plain disappearance is very real. Why such is considered an option of punishment in the first place is beyond me, and I believe, unconstitutional.

To analyze what I believe are to be some of the solutions to such problems, let's once more imagine that we're in the midst of a global pandemic. Let's assume that there has been some type of major bioterrorism event. The students can't simply up and move out to a new schooling system elsewhere, because everywhere has been affected the same. A weaponized strain of smallpox has been released on the US, and officials are doing everything in their power to keep some semblance of normalcy despite the mass death and devastation that is currently taking place.

If we were in such a situation (which is not that far off of an idea. Read Richard Preston's *Demon in the Freezer* for evidence), I think that there are a number of different approaches we could take – which while most certainly wouldn't be foolproof – would likely be some of the best options that we have available to us.

I think it's important to keep in mind that within this situation we need to keep physical contact, travel, and the like as minimal as possible. Thus, turning in any type of paper or notebook is likely not going to be a good idea.

As pointed out above, an *at-home* contingency plan is very important, but note that at-home doesn't have to mean *online*.

If we know that the students are only going to be out for a week or so (e.g. norovirus), perhaps the teachers could simply tell their students to read 2-3 chapters within their textbooks, and then have some type of written report, quiz, or test due for when everybody returns back to school. Such ensures that no technology is required, that the students have all the supplies that they need to succeed, and that the only obstacle standing between the student and their receiving a good grade will come from *the student's* own desire and effort.

However, I fully recognize that such a situation might only work for shorter durations. If we're talking about weeks to months, the situation is inherently different. This is where I believe that radio could be a novel means of public education. Within modern society, virtually everybody has access to a radio. They can easily be purchased from the Dollar General for those who don't have one as well. What if a county/region/state set aside twelve different frequencies to use for distance learning? There would be a frequency set aside for 1st grade, one for 2nd grade, and all the way to 12th. Students would easily be able to tune into their appropriate grade frequency and listen to 3rd grade math, reading, and spelling lectures complete with assignments that they could work on as the station was being played. It would be a stock lecture only requiring a pre-recorded teacher's lesson. All students within the region would have access to the same lecture, helping to avoid the logistical nightmare of every school having a separate frequency for each teacher to use.

Upon completion of whatever graded work the student needed to complete, the project could have a picture taken of it and sent via smartphone, could mail the project in, or drop the assignment off at a local "project drop box" once a month. This would help to ensure that all of the bases were covered so that there would be minimal contact between students, all students would be reachable, and there would be as minimal of a chance of children not being able to turn in their assignments as well. While such is currently not an option, I do believe that it has enough merit to consider thinking about.

"But how is this any different from the response that we saw with COVID from teachers and schools? Your approaches sound exactly the same?"

The difference is this:

Schools operated with bizarre policies throughout the COVID scam *despite* the data telling them they could do things normally. They continued to act as if paranoia was normal, and that one must take as many precautions as could be created in every situation all the time for eternity. For example, one school in Anchorage, Alaska was forcing pre-school children to kneel on pads on the floor all day rather than sit in the chairs at their desks. This allegedly was to "stop the spread." But that's not all.

In addition to those requirements, children were required to wear a mask all day, and had to bring all of their food, books, coats, and other school supplies to the classroom each day in *a 5-gallon bucket* because they were not allowed to use their lockers.[8] This is what I mean. How are any of these methods proven to combat disease? If anything, we're furthering the risk of injury to children by enacting such means. Lack of oxygen, orthopedic stress, and the forcing of preschoolers to awkwardly carry 5-gallon buckets full of books are all very real risks in such a situation.

If we're going to engage in public health policies that involve any form of school closure whatsoever, we need to ensure that what we're doing is supported by the true data. While I'm not inherently opposed to a school closing down or engaging in a distance learning format, to suddenly transition to such when there is no need is to create unnecessary hardships for a sizable portion of a population.

5

Lockdowns

"Food is power. We use it to change behavior. Some may call that bribery. We do not apologize." – Catherine Bertini, UN World Food Program Executive Director, 1997[1]

"The legislative has no right to absolute arbitrary power over the lives and fortunes of the people; nor can mortals assume a prerogative not only too high for men, but for angels, and therefore reserved for the Deity alone." – Sam Adams[2]

It was George Washington who compared government to fire. Both can be useful, but they can both be very terrible masters as well. It is hard to imagine an arena of life where this rings as true as within the range of public health. The 2020 coronavirus panic absolutely devastated the American economy. True, stock prices reached very high levels throughout the year, but I believe this came as a result of people being forced to buy products and services from major corporations (that had a presence on the stock market) who were still allowed to stay open while the mom-and-pop stores throughout the nation were either forced outright to close down or were given such stringent restrictions that there was no feasible and economic way that they could possibly stay in the black.

The author personally witnessed this firsthand. For three months I was deemed by my government to be an "unessential" worker. What does it mean when we have handed over power to government to determine who is unessential and who is not? As has been pointed out before, control over the production of wealth is control over human life itself. Why is one man's ability to feed and provide for his family deemed to be more important than another man's? Is this not at its very core a blatant violation of the principle that all men are created equal?

Perhaps some men truly matter more than others? How is an economy to operate in such a state? How is one to determine which career path to choose – which job will provide their family with uninterrupted income throughout disaster – if they are at the mercy of government officials who arbitrarily decide who is essential and who is not?

Such a man can never truly be sure that the career which he has chosen is in fact safe from a government enforced shutdown. If the government can hold a gun to a man's head and tell him that he is not allowed to work – that for his to do so is not "safe" – and this is due to no fault of his own – no mismanagement, no faulty practices, no sloppy work – but instead simply because the government deems it to be, then are we not at the mercy of tyrants?

Has history taught us nothing? Did we not witness the full ramifications of such a government position throughout the Holocaust? It was the Jews who were deemed to have useful occupations – who were deemed *essential* to the war effort – that were allowed to live (albeit, perhaps temporarily, and certainly in miserable conditions) while those who were deemed to be *unessential* were carted off to be gassed or shot. The control over who gets to live and who does not is a power that government does not possess outside of the scope of war or serious criminals. The right to life is one of the unalienable rights of man and is protected within the US

Constitution. To deprive a man of his right to provide is to deprive him of his right to eat – it is to deprive him of his right to life. Nobody on this earth has the authority to do such.

Adam Smith elucidates the concept in his book *Wealth of Nations*: "The statesman who should attempt to direct private people in what manner they ought to employ their capitals, would not only load himself with a most unnecessary attention, but assume an authority which could safely be trusted to no council and senate whatever, and which would nowhere be so dangerous as in the hands of a man who had folly and presumption enough to fancy himself fit to exercise it."[3]

There is no other way of looking at this. If you are to hold a man at the point of a gun anytime he attempts to work, you *are* directing the means by which he can employ his capital. You're telling him that he can't employ his capital whatsoever. The business owner who has established a coffee shop has invested a considerable sum into his storefront, benefits packages, equipment, beans, and the like. By refusing him access to his own property as well as his means to use it to provide for himself, you are mandating in which way he can employ his capital, and in which way he cannot. The man who believes he has the right to do such to others not only is oblivious to the individual needs of others but assumes a degree of power that was never his to take in the first place. It is blatant theft.

"Let's Destroy the Economy! Together!"

The lockdowns of 2020 will go down in history as one of the worst decisions that American politicians ever made – and even more one of the worse breaches of the American

Constitution that American politicians ever performed, *and that the American people tolerated*, as well. Let's take a further look at some of the reasons as to why.

According to the weekly Census Bureau data, as of July 17, 2020, approximately 12 million adults throughout America lived in households where the last rent payment had been missed, and about 23 million had little to no confidence that they would be able to pay their next rent bill. Many renters were left jobless due to the government-imposed lockdowns and forced reliance on unemployment benefits of $600 a week. As of the last week of June, more than 18 million people across the country were still applying for unemployment benefits. In order to correct a problem that government itself had created, government *then* decided to protect US renters via an eviction moratorium which prevented landlords from evicting tenants who did not pay their rents. This was initially set to expire on July 25, 2020. The city of Boston actually banned evictions throughout the rest of 2020.[4]

This in turn was an infringement on the rights of the landowner to their own property. If one buys a building with the purpose of living off of the proceeds of the rent, how can one meet *their* bills when the government decides that the tenants no longer have to pay? Is this not government confiscation of property? Is it not nationalization of all rental properties throughout the US? Does it not discourage future investors from ever becoming a landlord in the first place? Why invest in and begin a business where the government can step in at any time and decide that the customers don't have to pay? Why invest in a business where the customer is protected more than the investor?

From personal experience, I can speak to the fact that this eviction moratorium had a much larger rippling effect than any politician expected. I work as a locksmith, and one of our main sources of income derives from evictions. During evictions, we move in and change the locks to an apartment so that no squatting can continue. Due to the eviction moratorium, however, we completely lost that entire facet of our business, and that entire portion of our income. All because of government involvement.

Due to stringent COVID restrictions, other businesses throughout the US felt a similar squeeze. In fact, Yelp's July 22, 2020, Economic Average report showed that 60% of the 26,160 temporarily closed restaurants on its site had permanently shut. It's April report discovered that over 175,000 total businesses were closed in some capacity, and that just under 25% of those businesses were still open when July finally rolled around. As of July, 44% of 5454 temporarily closed bars and other nightlife venues were shut down for good as well.[5]

Further data from Yelp showed that as of July 10, permanent closures accounted for 55% of all closed businesses since March 1, 2020. The retail world was hit rather hard as well, with 26,119 total business closures and 12,454 permanent shutdowns within the retail market reviewed on Yelp as well. One can't help but wonder how many businesses were affected that *didn't* have a Yelp presence. Could the true numbers of permanent shutdowns potentially be exponentially higher?

It appears so. Azlo, a financial services company, conducted a survey at the end of May of the extent of the lockdowns and found that nearly *half* of all small business owners surveyed thought they would have to close their doors for good. A full 47% of those surveyed said that they anticipated shutting down in the future, and another 41% said that they were actually looking for full-time work elsewhere.[6] It probably need not be pointed out that when a business owner begins looking for work elsewhere, those who work under him necessarily must begin to do the same.

Further proof of the deleterious economic impact of lockdowns can be viewed from New York. As of August 10, 2020, the New York City Hospitality Alliance found that out of 500 restaurant owners, 83% said that they couldn't pay the entire rent of July. 37% actually paid no rent at all for that month.[7]

Come September, a NorthStar report found that 74% of US hotels expected to lay off more employees. A full two-thirds of hotel properties said that they wouldn't be able to last another six months at the current projected revenue and occupancy levels, while four out of five hotel properties within New York that were underpinning commercial mortgage bonds were on the verge of default. Of these hotels, 37.7% came to sit on a special watchlist that was created to warn investors of a mortgage's about to be transferred to debt collectors known as special servicers.

According to Vijay Dandapani, the chief executive of the Hotel Association of New York City, "the industry is really bleeding. It's not just on life support. It's comatose." He further went on to say that if just *half* of the city's 640 hotels survived the effects of 2020, that it would be a "great" outcome.[8]

Contrast this with Sweden's response to COVID-19. In Sweden throughout 2020, there weren't any lockdowns whatsoever. And as a result, Swedish companies by July 2020 were delivering profits well above what the market was expecting.[9] While Sweden does get a lot wrong, this does seem to be one arena of recent history where they made a correct decision. It's interesting to point out as well how it wasn't until well *after* the nation of Sweden and its response to COVID became a conservative talking point, that their numbers of *diagnosed* COVID cases began to increase.

As of mid-September 2020, however, Sweden was averaging one death per day from COVID, and this was due to a very liberal definition of what counted as a COVID death. The country hadn't had a day of double-digit deaths since July 19. All of the lockdown caused deaths, the economic destruction, the mental health crisis that other countries all seemed to experience – Sweden avoided all of it.[10]

Other foreign countries couldn't seem to get on board with Sweden's policy. Take Australia for example. By the beginning of August 2020, they had shut down the country for *another* six weeks. The premier of Victoria announced a state of disaster, introduced a nightly curfew, and banned virtually all outdoor trips. Further rules included: "Where you slept last night is where you'll need to stay for the next six weeks," and only one person per household being allowed to leave their homes once a day to pick up essential goods. The chosen person to leave the home also must stay within 5km of where they live.[11]

Are Lockdowns Justifiable?

So now that we have seen the very visible effects of what a lockdown does to the economy (which both indirectly and directly affects human health) as well as that of the human psyche, let us examine whether a government ever has the right to act with such destruction in the first place. We've touched on this briefly above, but let's give it a thorough investigation. One of mankind's most important rights is the right to own property. As Ayn Rand has pointed out, "Without property rights, no other rights are possible."[12]

If a man truly has the right to his own property, then he has the right to use and dispose of it as he seems fitting. To be told that one has the right to own property, but that they then cannot use that property in the manner in which it is intended is to own something in name only. Ayn Rand again points out, "Ownership without control is a contradiction in terms...It means that the citizens retain the responsibility of holding property, without any of its advantages, while the government acquires all the advantages without any of the responsibility."[13]

This is indeed what we saw throughout the entire COVID situation. To tell a business owner that he can no longer run his business and earn his income from the property on which his business resides is to rob him of his ability to use his rightfully owned property. What didn't change throughout this time was that the government still demanded their property taxes for the property and the bank still demanded their mortgage payments. The businessman owned a property in which he owned all of the risk – it was most certainly not the government who risked losing its entire income should his building foreclose – while the government still retained the advantage of taxing the property. In such a case, a man is made a slave without hope.

As patriot Samuel Adams said, "Now what liberty can there be where property is taken away without consent?"[2] The answer? None! How can one claim to live in or represent the Land of the Free when such blatant cases of theft are enacted against the American people? The fact of the matter is that "the control of the production of wealth is the control of human life itself."[14] Men were made slaves throughout 2020. The entire concept of lockdowns – of the division of men into "essentials" and "unessentials" – and all of the other ramifications of such are antithetical to American thought. Don't believe me? Check out what the Declaration of Independence has to say:

"We hold these truths to be self-evident: That all men are created equal: that they are endowed by their Creator with certain unalienable rights: that among these are life, liberty, and the pursuit of happiness: that, to secure these rights, governments are instituted among men, deriving their just powers from the consent of the governed: that whenever any form of government becomes destructive of these ends, it is the right of the people to alter or to abolish it, and to institute new government, laying its foundation on such principles, and organizing its powers in such form, as to them shall seem most likely to effect their safety and happiness."

If all are created equal, then we cannot forbid some from working. Life, liberty, and the pursuit of happiness are unalienable rights, correct? Then why did the US government deprive people of all three? And finally, was this forced policy of lockdown destructive towards life, liberty, and the pursuit of happiness?

Throughout the United States during this time millions across the country were forced into collecting unemployment insurance granted by the state. Leon Trotsky of Communist fame has pointed out the danger of such (albeit perhaps unwittingly): "In a country where the sole employer is the State, opposition means death by slow starvation. The old principle: who does not work shall not eat, has been replaced by a new one: who does not obey shall not eat."[15]

"But wait!" cries out the public health administrator. "This was all done in order to keep people *safe*! We *had* to lockdown the economy in order to stop the spread!"

I've already cited the research above which proves beyond a shadow of a doubt that lockdowns cause the death of economies and stop freedom more than they "stop the spread". If lockdowns worked there would never have been talk of *more* lockdowns after nations reopened. FA Hayek examines the logic behind this argument: "We could, of course, reduce casualties by automobile accidents to zero if we were willing to bear the cost – if in no other way – by abolishing automobiles. And the same is true of thousands of other instances in which we are constantly risking life and health and all the fine values of the spirit, of ourselves and of our fellow men, to further what we at the same time contemptuously describe as our material comfort. Nor can it be otherwise, since all our ends compete for the same means; and we could not strive for anything but these absolute values if they were on no account to be endangered."[16]

Perhaps we could eliminate all cases of drunk driving accidents by pushing through a new era of Prohibition. Perhaps we could eliminate all obesity by outlawing all food above 150 calories per serving. Perhaps we could eliminate all cases of rape by emasculating all men. Yet to talk of doing so is clearly both ridiculous and obscene. It is to talk of imposing slavery on others simply because *you* deem so to be best. It is a form of intellectual hubris in which the one making the decision has the notion that *their* idea is the correct one and must be *imposed* on a people *at all costs* – to keep them safe. Most certainly everyone believes that their own ideas are truth, and most certainly everyone does what they can to spread what they know to be true to others. But to argue against the freedom of another man – to argue for something that is both life-changing and incredibly destructive – for "the common good" is to work against good at every turn.

A lockdown and the separation of men into "essential" and "unessential" is to create a planned society. Hayek had this to say about such: "There [in a planned society] individuals will have to decide not whether a person is needed for a particular job but whether he is of use for anything, and how useful he is. His position in life must be assigned to him by somebody else."[17] This is exactly what happened. I was put on unemployment for three months because I was deemed by the government to be "unessential". My ability to provide for my family, to pay my mortgage, to make a dent in my student loans, to provide for my children, and to save for our future – all of it was deemed to be unessential by men who were working for the "common good". I noticed throughout this time though that the local city council, my state representatives, the governor, and the local public health officials were still allowed to work throughout this time, however. They still were permitted to ~~take~~ earn a paycheck after making it illegal for me to do the same. *Their* ability to pay their bills was apparently of more inherent worth than mine.

Adam Smith elucidated this concept within his masterpiece *The Wealth of Nations*. He said, "The patrimony of a poor man lies in the strength and dexterity of his hands; and to hinder him from employing his strength and dexterity in what manner he thinks proper without injury to his neighbor, is a plain violation of this most sacred property. It is a manifest encroachment upon the just liberty both of the workman, and of those who might be disposed to employ him. As it hinders the one from working at what he thinks proper, so it hinders the others from employing whom they think proper."[18]

And everyone who experienced likewise throughout the COVID situation only has those who were in office to blame. For "once government has embarked upon planning for the sake of justice, it cannot refuse responsibility for anybody's fate or position."[17]

Every man who lost his business, his home, his job, his family throughout the COVID situation as a result of a lockdown should seek his compensation from those who made the decisions, for it is they alone who bear fault. Such a notion should fill a politician's heart with fear. Did you lose your job? *It is the Department of Health's doing.* Did you lose your ability to feed your family? *It was your governor who robbed you of such.* Were you forced into government handouts? *Your city council did that to you.*

To those who argue that the lockdowns weren't really that bad, I believe Thomas Paine has the appropriate response in *Common Sense* when he argues against those who said the British invasion of America truly "wasn't that bad."

"But if you say, you can still pass the violations over, then I ask, Hath your house been burnt? Hath your property been destroyed before your face? Are your wife and children destitute of a bed to lie on, or bread to live on? Have you lost a parent or a child by their hands, and yourself the ruined and wretched survivor? If you have not, then you are not a judge of those who have. But if you have, and can still shake hands with the murderers, then you are unworthy the name of husband, father, friend, or lover, and whatever may be your rank or title in life, you have the heart of a coward, and the spirit of a sycophant."[19]

Furthermore, lockdowns only serve to increase the corruption within a nation, turning it from a nation of laws and morals, to a nation full of cheats and bribes. This comes logically. It is the natural result of such an action. As FA

Hayek points out for those living within a planned society: "...all our efforts directed toward improving our position will have to aim, not at foreseeing and preparing as well as we can for the circumstances over which we have no control, but at influencing in our favor the authority which has all the power."

How is it that a mega-corporation is allowed to remain open while the smaller businessman is forced to close down while held at the business end of a gun? Perhaps the businessman does not have the appropriate politician in his pockets? Hayek goes on: "As soon as the state takes upon itself the task of planning the whole economic life, the problem of the due station of the different individuals and groups must indeed inevitably become the central political problem. As the coercive power of the state will alone decide who is to have what, the only power worth having will be a share in the exercise of this directing power. There will be no economic or social questions that would not be political questions in the sense that their solution will depend exclusively on who wields the coercive power, on whose are the views that will prevail on all occasions."[17]

Adam Smith had this to say on the matter, "When the government has to decide how many pigs are to be raised or how many busses are to be run, which coal mines are to operate, or at what prices shoes are to be sold, these decisions cannot be deduced from formal principles or settled for long periods in advance. They depend inevitably on the circumstances of the moment, and, in making such decisions, it will always be necessary to balance one against the other the interests of various persons and groups. In the end somebody's views will have to decide whose interests are more important; and these views must become part of the law of the land, a new distinction of rank which the coercive apparatus of government imposes upon the people."[20]

Thus, we have the growth of state gangsterism. The growth of government oppression. The growth of cronyism. For as has been pointed out before, for the government to enforce tyrannical decrees it needs drastic punishment. That is the only way to get people to obey ridiculousness. If you want an individual to wear a mask all day which makes it difficult to breathe, you have to resort to drastic measures to get such to be complied with. If you want people to stay at home rather than go to work and provide for both their selves and their families, you have to threaten individuals with absolutely brutal punishment for going against such a natural (and just) desire.

"Just as the democratic statesman who sets out to plan economic life will soon be confronted with the alternative of either assuming dictatorial powers or abandoning his plans, so the totalitarian dictator would soon have to choose between disregard of ordinary morals and failure. It is for this reason that the unscrupulous and uninhibited are likely to be more successful in a society trending toward totalitarianism."[21]

But Do Lockdowns At Least Check Disease?

"Ok, ok. So lockdowns destroy economies. But if they stop disease, isn't the end worth the means? I mean, it doesn't do much good to be a rich dead guy, right? It's better to have lost your business and still be alive!"

Such may be the argument one would hear after coming to the conclusion that lockdowns cost millions their livelihood. But let us examine the matter. Is it correct? Do lockdowns actually prevent the spread of disease?

Science says no.

It was in January 2021 that infectious disease expert Professor Steven Riley said that the current data proved that the lockdowns throughout the UK didn't do a thing to stop COVID cases.[22]

Other scientists throughout the world found the same. The Great Barrington Declaration was a document signed by hundreds of doctors, scientists, epidemiologists stating that they knew lockdowns were ineffective in stopping the spread of disease and were actually destructive to health (aside from the negative consequences towards economies).

Yet over and over again what we saw was the silencing of any of those who presented evidence that was contrary to the official narrative. This was done underneath the argument that "the science is settled" despite the fact that the science was most certainly not "settled" and if anything, all of it pointed to the fact of lockdowns being a foolhardy and destructive means of getting nothing other than pain and suffering accomplished.

The Conclusion of the Matter

The message to those in charge of public health policy is clear: not only do you not have the *right* to forcibly lockdown a region, to do so doesn't even work in the first place. To think otherwise is to lead to "...the ultimate inversion: the stage where the government is free to do anything it pleases, while the citizens may act only by permission; which is the stage of the darkest periods of human history, the stage of rule by brute force."[23]

In no situation whatsoever should lockdowns be imposed on a people ever again in the future.

6

Forced Vaccinations

"But when the law, through the medium of its necessary agent – force – imposes a form of labor, a method or a subject of instruction, a creed, or a worship...it substitutes the will of the legislator for their own [the citizens'] will."
– Frederic Bastiat[1]
"In the part which merely concerns himself, his independence is, of right, absolute. Over himself, over his own body and mind, the individual is sovereign."
– John Stuart Mill[2]

The Tuskegee syphilis study was a landmark event in the world of medical ethics. There is scarce a soul alive within the US that would think that study was ethical. The forced infection of those men with syphilis so that the results could be studied is nothing short of murder. The same could be said for the heinous crimes against humanity that occurred throughout World War 2 by Nazi doctors and scientists those who found pleasure in treating human beings as guinea pigs – exposing them to unnecessary and undesired grotesque surgeries such as sewing multiple living human beings together, performing experiments on Jews with extremes of temperature, and the like.

The Nazis were also famous for discretely sterilizing those who they deemed to be a threat to the genetic pool of Germany. As Jews were asked to fill out forms at particular office's front desks, X rays were blasted at their genitals with such force that the victim would be left sterile just a few moments later and with no clue as to the reason why.[3]

Even within the US in the early 1900s we saw eugenics have an alive and well following. Hundreds were forcibly sterilized against their will through more invasive and painful procedures. Every medical textbook that you look at now which examines the ethics of such will leave one with no doubt that the world at large shudders when it thinks about what was forced upon others against their will, medically speaking. This is why informed consent matters. This is why the Nuremburg Code states that unauthorized medical treatments cannot be thrust upon an individual.

Yet these decisions to violate one's right to their own body – one's right of property, life, and liberty - were not something that happened just all of a sudden. A politician didn't just wake up one day and decide *this* – whatever 'this' may be – was what was going to happen. No, *instead*, what happened was decades worth of "research" proving this or that. Research had "proven" that Jews were an inferior race. Research had "proven" that Jews were harbingers of disease within a community. Research had "proven" this and that.

And it was a direct result of this research – of these scientists' conclusions – that public opinion was formed. Public opinion influences government policy, and once this occurred, it was only a matter of time before the most nightmarish of procedures were "legally" enacted against one's fellow man without his consent, and often without his knowledge as well.

The same applies for forced vaccinations. Man has a right to make his own decisions regarding his body. Though it has been widely perverted by abortion advocates, the phrase "My body, my choice" does have truth within it. To believe that one has the right to make a decision over somebody else's body is to show an incredible amount of hubris and pride in one's own self. It is to publicly state that *you* believe that you are better and wiser than Mr. Jones over there, and therefore have the right to make decisions for him that he does not want. There is most certainly the exception of those who are unable to voice their opinions on the matter. Those who have been involved in car crashes that have left them in a vegetative state, those with Alzheimer's, and the mentally retarded are going to need to have health decisions made for them in some instances.

But when we are talking about a human being who is in no way incapable of making his own decision, then what right do we have to force our will upon them when it comes to medical treatment? Obviously, there are going to be medical procedures that a doctor will deem to be too risky for such a patient, if there are typically a number of options available to do something such as fix a broken leg, and the doctor may deny the patient the choice of one of these treatments, but that is inherently different from forcing a medical procedure upon somebody who does not want it.

This is exactly what mandatory vaccinations amounts to. There are those within the US who are deathly afraid of firearms. Their fear may be completely unfounded, but to even have a firearm within the confines of their home would fill them with dread. Nobody can argue with the fact that the single woman with a firearm stands a much better chance against her home invader than does the single woman without one. Statistics actually show that she has a 99% chance of not being raped when she has a gun to fight back with! Without that gun, if she just cowers and begs, she has a 99% chance *of being raped.*[4] Yet despite this, we do not force these people to have a firearm in their home. The reason being that we understand that they have the right to choose for their own self. We may disagree with their decision – we may even think that it is foolish – but we do not have the right to make that decision for her. We could argue that the community as a whole would be safer if we were able to truthfully advertise at the neighborhood's gates that "This is an armed community", and that to be able to say such protects the health and welfare of the community as a whole, but does that change the fact that we are forcing somebody to engage in an action that is against their own judgment (and perhaps conscience as well)?

A man may believe that a vaccine is safe, effective, and a great boon to the public health of the community that he lives in. He may believe that if everyone within his community had such a vaccine, that it would better protect his own health. But does that give him the right to argue for the forcing of such a vaccine upon others who would rather not, regardless of what their personal reasonings might be? Absolutely not.

Though to the current reader it may appear as if I am solely arguing against the novel problem of the coronavirus shot, the fact is that the US has had a problem with mandatory vaccinations for years. One has been unable to work certain positions, attend particular schools, and more if they did not conform with the mandated vaccination against flu, HPV, chickenpox, measles, TB, and more for a very long time now. The forcing of a vaccine upon the American public is nothing new. For example, it was back during the swing flu pandemic that OSHA ruled employers could actually make a flu vaccination mandatory for employees.[5] So while this concept is not new, the coronavirus shot is the most present form of such, and as a result is weighs heavily on modern man's mind.

The problems with such a policy are numerous, however. For starters, when it's argued that being around other people is dangerous, don't violations of the First Amendment follow on the coattails of such an argument? If I say that unvaccinated people are spreaders of disease and don't deserve to be able to mix with society, then I am advocating for their being caged. Whether that prison is an actual jail or solely the walls of their own home, either way, I am arguing for imprisonment of others. I am arguing that they don't have the right to attend church, shop for groceries, meet with friends and family, and so on. *And all because of my own fear.* This is in direct violation of the First Amendment of the Bill of Rights.

But let us examine such the COVID shot even closer. Can it truly be argued that it is safe?

The research throughout 2020 did not appear to show so. A typical vaccination within the US requires ten years of research before it is approved by the FDA (provided the research shows the vaccine safe and effective). The COVID-19 vaccine had less than a year. It's not comforting when one realizes that due to the FDA's Public Readiness and Emergency Preparedness Act (PREP), all vaccine manufacturing companies were granted protection from all legal action should something go wrong with those who are vaccinated as well. AstraZeneca was granted similar protection in England.[6]

Would you fly in a plane in which Boeing had been granted immunity from any legal actions taken against it for? What about a car? Would you drive in a Ford in which Ford was not to be held liable for anything *whatsoever* going wrong with the car? Perhaps the wheels could all fall off once you reached 65 mph. Oh well! They were granted legal immunity! Would you go to see a doctor for surgery if right before he operated, he told you, "Just to let you know, there's zero liability for me here if I screw you up."? If he cut off the wrong limb, leaving you in a wheelchair for the rest of your life, there'd be nothing you could do about it! Odds are that your answers to any of the above questions would be a resounding "NO". So, why do we see people so adamant about jumping in line to get a brand-new shot?

"But surely they tested these shots! They wouldn't let something blatantly dangerous out onto the market!"

Well, let us take a look. For starters, it was said that the vaccine could actually cause people to be more likely to die from the virus due to something called vaccine induced immune enhancement.[7] That's quite lovely, is it not?

Australia's University of Queensland actually canceled further development of their COVID vaccine in December of 2020 after several trial participants ended up giving false positives for HIV.[8] What exactly is going on in the human body in these situations that is causing that to happen?

The US FDA admitted around the same time that two participants in the Pfizer COVID vaccine phase 3 trials had died. Brazil halted a Sinovac trial as well after a participant died. A Philadelphia priest participated in the Moderna trial, dying not long after receiving his second dose.[9] The AstraZeneca COVID vaccine faced its fair share of problems as well. It was put on hold during September 2020 after suspected serious adverse reactions in a UK trial participant.[10]

And death wasn't the only potential risk one faced when getting a COVID-19 shot in 2020. The US government actually cautioned women of child-bearing age against getting the vaccine. They were told that they should avoid becoming pregnant until at least two months after being COVID vaxxed. This was because at the time there was zero testing done on the side effects of such a vaccine on lactation, fertility, or pregnancy.[11] Other authorities cautioned men that they may want to consider freezing their semen before getting the vaccine.[12]

Within the UK, regulators cautioned those with a history of allergic reactions to either food or medicine away from getting the COVID vax. This came after two NHS workers experienced allergic reactions (referred to as "anaphylactoid reactions") to the new Pfizer vaccine. It should be noted that an anaphylactoid reaction tends to involve a skin rash, breathlessness, and sometimes a drop in blood pressure.[13]

Oh. Well, that sounds nice. There's nothing like a nice precipitous drop in blood pressure and a little breathlessness to help you move your day along. And as if that wasn't bad enough later reports showed people throughout the world ending up becoming magnetic after receiving their COVID shot. Numerous videos began to surface on the internet early 2021 as people learned that they could stick magnets, pieces of metal, and even cell phones against their body and they would stick in place.[14] This wasn't the only side effect experienced by people though. Within the US, the CDC keeps a list known as the Vaccine Adverse Event Reporting System (VAERS). This list is kept for various shots so that people can gauge how dangerous/what the risks may be to getting injected with something.

With the COVID shot, CDC data showed that more people had died within the past 6 months of COVID shots because of COVID shots than had died in the prior 20 years from shots *combined*. That should be a cause of hesitation for anybody. Furthermore, it's believed that only 1% of adverse events are actually ever reported to the VAERS database in the first place.[15]

Yet despite the plethora of evidence showing that a COVID vaccination may not be the wisest idea ever thought up, and despite *any* vaccine being made mandatory being a blatant human rights violation, countries around the world jumped on the bandwagon together in the effort to make it a crime to refuse the COVID shot.

The USA

Within the US an Operation Warp Speed was created with the goal of vaccinating as many Americans as possible. General Gus Perna was in charge of the operation and had this to say: "Upon emergency use authorization, all of America must receive [the] vaccine within 24 hours."[16] As of June 2021, that has yet to happen, but it's the principle behind the policy that needs to be reviewed. Further time within the US revealed that the FBI had created a vaccine passport that it was going to push upon the American people, and that the FBI itself would punish those who created fake vaccine passports.[17]

Oregon later became the first state of the Union that required constituents to show proof of vaccination to go out in public.[18]

Great Britain

Britain was something of an enigma throughout the COVID-19 situation when it comes to mandatory vaccination. During November of 2020, Prime Minister Boris Johnson said that the UK would not mandate the COVID vaccine.[19]

However, less than a month later The Sunday Times reported that Britain was in the process of utilizing a secretive and elite military intelligence agency – which had been used in the hunt against the Taliban and al-Qaeda and with psyops teams in the past - to seek out "anti-vaccine militants" and related "propaganda content" throughout cyberspace. It's long been no secret that freedom of speech does not exist within Britain (or anywhere in Europe for that matter), but this was a new degree of infringement on basic human rights.[20]

Imagine having a military team sent after you because you have said something that the government doesn't like. Such sounds reminiscent of Nazi Germany, fascist Italy, or Russia, does it not?

Canada

Canada was an absolutely horrific place to live throughout the COVID panic. There were multiple reasons why – chief of which being that their president deserves to be shipped one-way to Russia – but their stance on mandatory vaccination was paramount as well. During December of 2020, Ontario's Chief Medical Officer said, "What may be mandatory, is proof of vaccination, in order to have latitude and freedom to move around without wearing personal protective equipment." He also stated that though Canada couldn't force someone to take a vaccine they *could* make things as difficult as possible for you.[21]

"We're Not FORCING You. You're Free to Leave..."

This raises the problem of using cloudy logic to say that you're not forcing something on somebody, you're just going to make their life miserable. And that is one of the problems with the idea of a mandatory vaccine is that it is likely that many governments won't *explicitly* force people to get the desired vaccine. Some will, and I believe most *will* use force in the very near future, but in the interim, I believe this is what's going to happen.

What they *will* do is make life as unpleasant as possible unless you *do* get the vaccine. Though there may be no law stating that everyone within the country must get a particular vaccine, there very well could be a great number of employers, storefronts, churches, and forms of transportation that won't permit you to utilize their services if you do *not* have the vaccine. John Stuart Mill had this to say on the matter:

"When society is itself the tyrant – society collectively, over the separate individuals who compose it – its means of tyrannizing are not restricted to the acts which it may do by the hands of its political functionaries. Society can and does execute its own mandates: and if it issues wrong mandates instead of right, or any mandates at all in things with which it ought not to meddle, it practices a social tyranny more formidable than many kinds of political oppression, since, though not usually upheld by such extreme penalties, it leaves fewer means of escape, penetrating much more deeply into the details of life, and enslaving the soul itself.

Protection, therefore, against the tyranny of the magistrate is not enough: there needs protection also against the tyranny of the prevailing opinion and feeling; against the tendency of society to impose, by other means than civil penalties, its own ideas and practices as rules of conduct on those who dissent from them; to fetter the development, and, if possible, prevent the formation, of any individuality not in harmony with its ways, and compel all characters to fashion themselves upon the model of its own."[22]

I'm of the belief that one of the best means to counter against such is through the availability of a free press. Spoken and written word does change minds. There is no doubt about that. How many college students do you know who have entered their state-run university innocent, patriotic, and loving, only to exit a hate-filled, blue-haired, communist? Words matter. Likewise, money matters as well. Provided a free market is being run, and I have the opportunity to refuse somebody business because they are not people I like, I am able to vote with my dollar. I can now go to the coffee shop across the street instead, spending my money there. When enough people do this, they're able to cause the offending coffee shop to consider changing its policy (or perhaps it will be run out of business). The third way to fight this is to ensure that the populace at large is well-versed in the subject of human rights. Provided that people are knowledgeable enough to know what is a violation of human rights and what is not, they'll be better able to see where they're being wicked or not.

The outcome of government or society public health mandates is in effect the same either way though. It's interesting to note the arguments used for such a purpose. One will be told that a private business has the right to refuse service to whoever they like. However, such a standard is never held bilaterally. If one were to refuse service to blacks, gays, liberals, or feminists there would quickly be public outcry. Meanwhile, it's perfectly acceptable to deny interviews to whites, target conservatives with the IRS, or tell whites they can't get particular scholarships solely because of their skin color.

There are specific laws within the US protecting such people groups from discrimination. Within the US, you can't tell a man in a wheelchair that he's not allowed to come into your business because he's in a wheelchair. In fact, the American's With Disabilities Act actually forces you to accommodate such a customer by having hallways and doorways that are a particular width. However, there doesn't seem to be any protection for those who refuse vaccination. Imagine if you will, refusing service to those who aren't circumcised. You would have to ask each person as they come through your front doors for proof of circumcision (in the form of an ID card). Those who weren't circumcised, you wouldn't let through your doors. Is not somebody else's health information *their* information? Is it not private? Why do we completely throw privacy to the wind when it comes to vaccination?

Most certainly, I understand the reasoning behind refusing service to somebody who is actively sick. If a man comes into your store looking like death warmed over, hacking violently, runny nose, and with an incredibly hoarse throat, I do understand somebody not wanting to work with them. But how can you run a business operating under the assumption that *everybody* is a leper and that they must be treated accordingly?

Such is the case with Qantas. In November of 2020, Qantas CEO Alan Joyce said, "We are looking at changing our terms and conditions to say for international travelers, that we will ask people to have the vaccination before they get on the aircraft." No vaccination, no flying with Qantas.[23]

Other companies (and politicians) have followed suit with such ideals. Ticketmaster stated that future events will not allow customers to enter the stadium or auditorium unless they show proof of vaccination. New Jersey Senator Joseph Vitale (D) said that the COVID vaccine needs to be made mandatory for all school-age children as a condition for entering school with no exceptions.[24]

Who Do Children Belong To? The State? Or the Parent?

Does a parent have the right to determine whether or not their own children should be vaccinated for a particular illness or does that right belong to the state? It doesn't take much forethought to understand that the answer to this question helps to determine who the child really belongs to in the first place.

In June 2020, Colorado pushed through a bill that reduces the exemptions on mandatory vaccinations for public school children. If a parent wanted a different vaccination schedule from what the state of Colorado demands, the parent must then be registered for and attend an online "education" module and then submit a certificate of completion from the re-education class in order to receive the state-sanctioned vaccine exemption. The bill also forces doctors throughout Colorado to give vaccinations with no exemptions, *even if the doctor believes that vaccinating a child for a particular illness would cause more harm than good.* This means that even if the doctor knew that giving a particular vaccine to a child with an egg allergy could be dangerous, he would be required to give it. Allergic reactions are therefore legally mandated by the state of Colorado.

Furthermore, the bill requires public schools to publicly report what percentage of their students are either vaccinated or exempt from vaccination – and schools are given goals of 5% or less of their students being exempt. How exactly schools are to "encourage" students to not attempt to get vaccine exemptions is unclear. I'm sure you can imagine how such would play out.

Colorado's not alone in this either. New York, California, West Virginia, Maine, and Mississippi all deny vaccine exemptions based off of religious belief as well. Because apparently the state matters more than your private convictions. Illinois is attempting to push through similar laws as of this writing as well.[25] This is a blatant violation of the First Amendment. You are no longer allowed to worship and act as you please, because now you have become the property of the state. Your body is no longer your own. And for those who *refuse* to take a mandatory vaccination, the consequences are always severe. They have always been so in the past, and they will continue to grow even more horrific in the future.

Shouldn't Vaccines Work?

If one is going to get a vaccine, it would be nice if it actually did what it was advertised to do, would it not? Would you go and get a chickenpox shot if it didn't actually protect you from chickenpox? No?

Would it surprise you to find that people thought the polar opposite when it came to the COVID-19 shot? As of June of 2020, a Chinese study published in Nature Medicine had found that the antibodies produced by COVID patients actually fades relatively quickly when compared to the fading period of other infection antibodies. Subjects within the study actually saw their antibodies to COVID-19 drop by more than 70% over a period of *eight weeks*.[26] A UK study discovered similar findings. A group of researchers at King's College London found that antibody levels to COVID-19 peak three weeks after symptoms appear, and then begin to fade significantly. In some cases, the antibodies faded away completely.[27]

Would you get a shot that only lasts for eight weeks? This would mean the mandating of regular booster shots, would it not?

In late November of 2020, AstraZeneca announced that its new adenovirus-vector vaccine (ChAdOx1) was around 70% effective. Keep in mind that that's not a passing grade in school. SVB Leerink analyst George Porges analyzed the AstraZeneca's published study and found that the results were published without enough data on safety. The design of the trials for ChAdOx1 didn't appear to match the minimum criteria for such according to the Food and Drug Administration.[28] However, as 2021 continued to roll along it appears that this widescale acknowledgement of COVID shot ineffectiveness was something that the American public was just supposed to roll with.

We were told that though the vaccine didn't keep you from getting COVID (there were thousands of cases throughout the US of people being diagnosed with COVID after receiving their shot), that it did keep you from getting terribly sick if you did get COVID. I personally know of an individual who told me that it was a good thing her three relatives in India had all gotten the COVID shot because they had all gotten severely sick with COVID shortly afterwards. "Imagine if they hadn't gotten their shot!" Wait a minute. So they got the shot, and fell violently ill shortly afterwards? Am I the only one who sees a problem with such?

This wasn't just an isolated incidence either. This was yet another difficult to swallow pill that the MSM continually shoved down Americans' throats: the notion that getting violently ill after getting the COVID shot was normal and a sign that the shot was working. I am personally aware of people who basically lost their ability to move for several days post-shot, of people who spent months with violent chills post-shot, of entire businesses/schools having to shut down after offering a COVID shot clinic on-site because so many people ended up sick, and *you* likely have experienced similar reports.

Why are people getting so violently ill from the COVID shot? Why did the miscarriage rate skyrocket after the COVID shot was released? Why were there more vaccine-related deaths within less than half a year post-COVID shot than there were in the past 20 years combined? Why mandate that everybody get a vaccine if *you're* already protected by your vaccine? If you're good, why must I also get the shot? Does it not work?

These are all valid questions that millions throughout the US had in 2021. And now for the crux of the matter, under no circumstances whatsoever should a vaccine ever be made mandatory by the state.

7

Should You Trust a Government that Must Convince You?

This discussion on mandatory vaccines – particularly ones that don't work – brings me to my next point: social convince you? I really believe that one of the most telling things about a policy is the degree of work it takes for such to be forced upon the people. If a great majority of the populace is against a given policy, does that not say something about the inherent nature the policy? Does it not say something for those who still attempt to force it down the throats of those citizens whom they are supposed to serve?

Such was the case with COVID-19. Yale University actually collaborated with the US government in a study titled "Persuasive messages for COVID-19 vaccine uptake: a randomized controlled trial, part 1" to help determine the best message to "persuade" Americans to get the COVID-19 vaccine.[1]

This reeks somewhat of studying LSD to determine how one can manipulate somebody while they are under the influence, does it not? When a government is studying ways in which to *manipulate* the public at large to go through with something that they would ordinarily find absurd, you can rest assured that tyranny is on the way. If you have to be manipulated to make a decision, it's likely to be a decision you would never have made of your own accord.

This leads me to the four-step process that governments use to convince their populace to go along with some type of action. I believe that there is firm evidence of all four steps within the United States ever since the COVID panic began in January 2020.

Step 1: Propaganda

Of course, first and foremost is using propaganda. One would like to believe that they are completely immune to the effects of such, but the fact of the matter is that propaganda works. If you expose even the most intelligent of individuals to effective propaganda long enough, you eventually just might end up with a brainwashed man with a lot of credentials behind his name. Joseph Goebbels demonstrated such throughout Nazi Germany. Propaganda was a large part of the reason why the Holocaust was ever able to happen in the first place.

By the time that the shot came around, Americans had been subjected to a full year of propaganda by the entire mainstream media regarding how dangerous and prevalent COVID was. It's a large part of the reason why so many people were convinced to take the COVID shot. However, there are other ways in which a government may "convince" somebody to take a particular action. When propaganda doesn't do the trick, the next step is to use public shaming.

Step 2: Public Shaming

For the most part, the government never even has to do this part. Once propaganda has firmly taken root throughout the majority of a nation, the citizens will do this part for them. By this point in the process, the large segments of society have become fully convinced that to engage in a certain behavior is the only wise choice and that those who do not do so are fools. And not just any fools, but dangerous fools as well.

Emotions have already been stoked to a high degree by the propaganda, and those who have swallowed it will have been successfully swayed into thinking that those who don't follow the same government-endorsed beliefs or actions are a danger to society. This causes the brainwashed to believe that "something out to be done" about those people. It is a result of this opinion that they're willing to engage in mockery and other acts of public shaming that they may not otherwise engage in under normal circumstances.

For proof of such, consider the wide range of negative interactions you likely had throughout your own community were you an anti-masker/pro-freedom throughout the entire COVID panic. I personally witnessed numerous screaming matches (which were always started by the human rights violator – the masker), unceasing name calling of those who didn't comply with COVID regulations, and the like. While there was most certainly my own anecdotal experience, there was public shaming at the government level as well throughout the US during this time.

Exhibit A would be Houston's Democratic mayor, Sylvester Turner. It was in June of 2020 that he floated the idea of creating a "board of shame" for city businesses that violated Harris County's mask mandate. As of that time, the mask mandate required that all businesses enforce mask usage for staff *and customers* while indoors. Turner had this to say, "I do think it's important for people to know who's being a good citizen, and who's not." He went on to say, "We want people to be good partners and good citizens. If you are not, you need to go on the board of shame."[2]

Masking wasn't the only situation where public shaming was used. I had numerous people criticize my refusal to take the COVID shot. These were people who changed the subject of conversation to ask me if I was getting the shot or not. When I said no, I was then told all of the reasons that I was in the wrong. That I "wasn't doing what I was supposed to." That I had others to think about, and which I was neglecting to do so. How can this be viewed as anything other than public shaming? And while peer pressure works in high school (where this type of behavior is scary to me when it comes to COVID shots – convincing a kid to take the shot because all of his 'friends' are making fun of him), I don't think it's as effective as some of the other steps within this process.

Step 3: Bribes

After public shaming comes bribes. This often comes in the form of tax incentives/subsidies for those who wouldn't normally engage in certain activities. For example, American farmers are routinely given subsidies to grow corn and soybeans. Sometimes they're given subsidies to let their crop rot in the field so that prices for that particular commodity will stay artificially elevated. Some cities have used gun buyback programs to allegedly "reduce gun violence" within a community.

To the best of my knowledge, public health was largely immune to bribes until 2021. While there have always been medical studies that would pay participants to try a new medication/treatment, this was more on the medical side of the spectrum than it was on the public health side (there is a difference that public health professors are rather adamant about). If we're talking about activities and policies that affect the health of a population as a whole, this author doesn't remember ever hearing about any form of bribe prior to 2021's use of bribes to get people to get the COVID shot. This isn't to say that such *did not* take place in the past, it's just that I'm not aware of it.

Lotteries began to actually pop up throughout the US in 2021 where *taxpayer dollars* were used to pay out massive cash prizes to those who got their COVID shot. West Virginia gave trucks, guns, lifetime hunting and fishing licenses, while California, Colorado, Maryland, New Jersey, and other states seemed to mainly stick with massive cash payouts.[3] And all at the taxpayer's expense. If you live in one of those states, your money was taken out of your hand so that others could receive a fortune to engage in an activity that you don't believe in. Such is disgusting, theft, and tyrannical.

The problem though, was that it appeared as if it was working. Within Ohio in particular, 3.2 million people got the COVID shot after the introduction of the lottery. This was *months* after these people had been eligible for the shot as well.[4] The lottery worked (that is, if the reported numbers are true. There's a history of false data here, so we must take what we hear with a grain of salt.). It coaxed reluctant people to engage in an activity they otherwise would never have gone along with. And I highly doubt that Ohio is an isolated case. If it worked there, there's no reason to believe that the shot lotteries aren't working in other states as well. At least to an extent.

What happens when a government finds that bribes no longer work?

Step 4: Force

It is then that the government resorts to force. After propaganda has mobilized the masses, after they've begun to build their public fury and become desensitized to public shaming, after it's found that bribes only get you so far, it is then that the government resorts to brutal force. While in some instances (such as masking), government force was moved to right after Step 1, I believe that the mandatory COVID shot is following the traditional four-step process.

As such, I believe that it is only a matter of time until men with guns and armored vehicles are sent to areas to enforce vaccination amongst the unwilling. While as mentioned above, I believe that the "we're not forcing you. Just making your life miserable" argument will be used initially, sooner or later, it will turn to the use of force. Do not let it come to you as a surprise.

8

Reasons to Lock People Up

"Man's rights can be violated only by the use of physical force." – Ayn Rand[1]

It has been pointed out that the average American citizen commits three felonies every single day.[2] This is the problem of what legal experts call "overcriminalization". It is the reason that an audit by the IRS is truly terrifying. You can be as conscious as possible to do everything in your power to follow the law, but there is undoubtedly going to be some obscure law that you were not aware of – in fact that you had never even had told you – and if found guilty of such, you will face the full weight of the law. You will be slapped about with the tagline, "Ignorance of the law is no excuse, sir."

While in some cases that is true – murder is inherently understood worldwide to be morally repugnant – even if you didn't know it was illegal, ignorance in such a case is no excuse. In others though, not so much. Imagine a child playing on a grassy bank at a wedding reception at a hoity toity historical home. He's four years old and having the time of his life. That's when venue host comes out and yells at the little kid to quit playing on the bank. Embarrassed, the child runs amidst the crowd to his father.

It's not long until the little boy is back playing on the bank though. Rolling down it is a new discovery of his, and he's enjoying every minute. The reception host sees the little boy once more, and visibly angered once more yells for the boy to get off the bank. The father is nearby this time and comes over to see what is going on. "This is the second time I've had to tell your child to get off of the bank!" the host gusts. The father looks down at the boy and asks, "Did she tell you to get off the bank before?"

Looking up mournfully, the little boy squeaks out a 'yes'.

"Alright," says the father. "Come with me."

Holding the little boy by the hand, the father walks back to his truck. It's there that he puts the child over his knee and spanks him. The boy is in tears as his father cradles him close to his chest.

"You have to listen when adults tell you something, kiddo," he says.

The little boy responds, "Daddy, what's a bank?"

Sometimes, ignorance of the law *is* an excuse. Anything outside the realm of natural law (e.g. don't murder, steal, destroy property, etc.) is not going to be as well-known of a law. While functioning adults need to understand the laws in the region that they live in, if they go to visit a neighboring state, the odds they're going to know all of the different laws is virtually zero. Even in their own locale, the odds of their knowing every law on the books is going to be infinitesimally small. I would argue that even a local lawyer couldn't do it.

The point is, ever since we've let our government become bloated and massive there are always going to be laws that you are breaking *without ever knowing it.*

This is one of the reasons that privacy is so vital to freedom. The more you look, the more you find. This basic principle applies to a great number of situations in life. The joke within orthopedic clinics is that if you want an excuse to get surgery, get an MRI. You're bound to find a tear *somewhere.* Law enforcement can be used to do the very same thing. Send enough health inspectors and detectives to the scene and they're bound to find *something* being done that's been deemed illegal. Privacy makes for a fantastic defense in such a case.

This is largely caused by overcriminalization. If you make everybody a criminal then you can get rid of people anytime they become inconvenient, burdensome, or dangerous to you as a politician. It's the perfect weapon. And the problem with all of these laws is that many (perhaps the great majority) don't even have a right to exist in the first place. What do I mean by this?

It is hard to imagine a realm of man's life that is more likely to be used in a totalitarian and unconstitutional manner than the field of public health. When the public health official is permitted to make laws without any checks and balances, you truly have a totalitarian in your midst. The reason that the US is comprised of the executive, judicial, and legislative branches is so that one cannot become more powerful than the other. The reason that we have a very specific set of procedures to follow – as written within the Constitution – for laws to be passed, is so that they *cannot* be arbitrarily passed by single entities without any form of checks and balances whatsoever.

Imagine the terror that comes from living under the reign of an all-powerful king. Anything he says goes, and perchance you do something to tick him off, your very life could be forfeit. History has shown this over and over again. Look at the story of Esther within the Bible. It only took one man's actions – Mordecai's – to convince one other man – Haman, trusted adviser to the king – that the entire Jewish race needed to be exterminated. This was all because Mordecai wouldn't bow to Haman. What is to happen should one inadvertently offend such a tyrant (or his friends)? The end result could be terrifying. There are doubtless countless other examples that you can think of.

Yet despite our basic understanding of such – despite our understanding that dictators are dangerous – that we have no desire to live under a Stalin, a Lenin, a Castro, a Zedong – we still have allowed such men and women to be given free reign within our very own locales. These are the public health officers.

Public health offices are not held responsible for any of the decisions that they make. There is no system of checks and balances for them. They simply issue decrees, and if such are not followed, then there are potentially grave consequences.

Now examine what could happen should two children get into a fight at school. One child's father is a public health officer, while the other's is a gym owner. Is it too far-fetched of an idea to think that a fickle and petty man would never use his power to harass another? If there were a virus scare, would this not give the perfect pretext for getting back at the man who is deemed to have a troublesome son? I am most certainly not saying that this is what happened throughout the nation in 2020 to gym owners, but I think it is naïve and foolish to believe that such is not possible.

We *have* seen examples of such. Why else would a public health official show up to a church on a weekday and cite them for violating health codes, when they have in fact followed all of the regulations to a tee? Is this perhaps because the official has some personal vendetta against Christianity or Semitism in general? Perhaps such an action is their own "fight" against what they deem to be an evil of society?

Throughout 2020 overcriminalization of the American public (and of the citizens of the rest of the world as well) was taken to the extreme. Public health officers were given seemingly limitless powers to impose whatever regulations they desired. And this was typically done without any logic behind the decision whatsoever. Any logic backed *by science* for a desired public health outcome, that is. The only logical reason much of the American people were turned into criminals throughout 2020 by public health officials likely has more to do with communism than it had to do with any true public health rationale.

How else does one explain a paddle boarder in California being arrested while out on the water for violating a stay-at-home order? How much more socially distanced can one be than being out alone on a board in the middle of the ocean? That poor guy actually had a police ship sent after him. The charges against him were a $1000 fine and/or six months in jail. Yes, you read that correctly. Six months in jail for riding a paddle board at the beach. And why? Because COVID regulations made such illegal.[3]

He was by no means the sole victim of such laws either. And they truly were severe. There is no denying that, and public health officials wanted *even more* power to enforce their "laws" than they actually got as well. This should be a prime evidence of power creating a lust for more power.

For example, Dr. Muntu Davis, a health officer for Los Angeles County said, "If it were up to me, anybody not wearing a mask when they are out in public would be arrested. That's an act of domestic terrorism and should be treated like one."[4]

One comes to wonder when exactly it became a crime to show one's face in public. It's strange to come to a time in history where people believe they are morally superior because they refuse to show their face in public. It's too bad that they don't keep their voice hidden as well. It's unfortunate that Dr. Davis, a doctor, isn't knowledgeable enough about infectious diseases to know why public masking is a terrible idea. His statement seems to be proof that he is ignorant regarding the presence of N95 masks as well. Such is a shame and a pathetic excuse for a doctor. Wouldn't a better example of domestic terrorism be tyrants imposing their unlawful will upon the people they are supposed to serve? What should be done to those people?

This desire to impose severe punishments on those who didn't comply with public health official doctrine wasn't isolated to just California, however. Englewood, Colorado issued an emergency order *requiring* citizens to wear masks. These emergency mandates seemed to begin around the beginning of July and quickly spread across the country from there. Those who did not were at risk of up to a year in prison. According to the emergency order, all citizens older than five years old were required to mask themselves in public. The first offense was a fine of $15. The second offense was $25. After that, there was a maximum penalty of $2650 or up to 360 days in prison.[5]

How exactly $2650 equates to a year in prison is beyond me, but it was 2020. Nothing had to make sense. It's interesting to note as well that in Colorado, one can be sentenced to jail for a year for forgery, theft, and failure to register as a sex offender as well.[6]

Who in their right mind would equate somebody who doesn't wear a mask in public with somebody who is a sex offender? Yet that is what we saw throughout 2020 consistently. Sharon Hurt of the Nashville Metro Council had a similar opinion for those who refuse to wear face masks, believing that should they do so and transmit COVID to somebody else that they should actually be found guilty of either murder or attempted murder.[7] What are the two possible punishments for murder in the United States? Execution or lifetime imprisonment. By extension, was she not saying that either of those two options should be considered for those who refuse to mask? That she wants you dead? That she wants you locked away forever?

The scary thing about such a prospect is that contact tracing isn't always an exact science. Sometimes people get sick with things and we truly have no clue where the infection could have possibly come from. What if that were the case, yet you were deemed to be the cause of somebody else's infection? What if the other person actually had a false-positive test for COVID? Now you're charged with attempted murder for a crime that you didn't actually commit.

Other locations within the US parroted this type of behavior.

- In Beverley Hills, California, not wearing a mask would cost you $100 for the first offense, $200 for the second, and $500 the third.
- Houston's mayor Sylvester Turner announced a $250 fine on those who refused to comply with his mask mandates.
- New Mexico had a $100 fine for not wearing a mask
- Washington DC fined people up to $1000 for not wearing a mask
- West Hollywood charged $300 for a first offense of not wearing a mask
- Glendale, California charged $400 for a first offense, $1000 for a second offense, and $2000 for a third offense of going maskless in public
- Numerous Californian beaches charged $100 fines.[8]

Surprisingly, even South Dakotans fell prey to this mode of thinking. In September 2020, Reed Bender was removed from a school board meeting – that was meeting in regards to public opposition to the district's mask mandate – for not wearing a mask. Because he refused to wear a mask at a First Amendment protected event where he was voicing his reasoning why forced mask wearing was unconstitutional, Superintendent Joe Graves called the cops on Reed who then pulled a taser on Bender and threatened to use it.

Here we have a law-abiding American citizen exercising Constitutionally protected rights having a taser pulled on him and being escorted out of a taxpayer funded building because he refused to listen to the dictatorial mandates of one man. Did that man have the authority to issue a mask mandate in the first place?

Board member Kevin Kenkel even went so far to say, "Even if 75% said we don't want masks, I would still vote in favor of masks."[9] Remember this is a voted in representative! These are people that are supposed to represent the best interests of the people! How can you reach the mental verdict that you as a politician are smarter than the people that you are supposed to serve? Even if 75% of them tell you that they don't want X, *you* know better, *you* are smarter, and thus, *your* will needs to be enforced on the people. If they don't like it they better shut up or else you're going to send cops with tasers, batons, and pistols after them.

North Korea actually took this type of logic to its full culmination. Radio Free Asia reported on December 4, 2020 that a citizen of North Korea had been *publicly executed* after violating COVID lockdown laws there. Sharon Hurt, rejoice. At this time North Korea's dictator, Kim Jong Un, had lockdowned entire cities and counties, canceled culture events, and even stopped travel between provinces. Other reports stated that a citizen "smuggler" had been executed in Ryongchon County on November 28, as well as potentially a currency exchange broker in the capital who allegedly broke quarantine laws. In addition to executing its own citizens, North Korea has given orders to its border soldiers to shoot anyone who comes within a half mile of the border for any reason whatsoever. To further assist in their quarantine efforts, they've placed landmine fields throughout the border line as well.[10]

And this is the logical culmination of such a philosophy. Make no mistake. This should terrify those who live elsewhere. For if this truly is the logical culmination of all the stepping stones of being "legally" allowed to cover peoples' faces in public, of robbing them of their ability to earn a living, of being able to lock them in their houses, of forcing substances into their bodies, how long will it be before similar policies – executions – are put into place in *your* country?

North Korea isn't the only foreign country that has criminalized its own citizens due to COVID violations. Canada followed suit rather quickly. Adam Skelly opened his BBQ restaurant in Toronto on November 24,2020 only to be ordered by the Toronto Public Health Department to close later in that same day. Despite this, he opened his restaurant again on Wednesday. Early Thursday morning before he got there, authorities responded by changing the locks *to Adam Skelly's own restaurant*. How about we call this what it rightfully is? Vandalism. What would be the consequences if somebody did the same to the local police station, city hall, or the mayor's house? Why is it ok to do it to a citizen?

When Adam showed up to work later that morning he was *also* met by a significant police presence. He still tried to reopen his restaurant despite this, and was then promptly arrested, being charged with intent to obstruct police, *holding an illegal gathering*, and trespassing *on his own property*. How one can do this is beyond me. He was released on bail 30 hours later but was *then* given the condition that he couldn't post about his experience on social media. One has to wonder what type of government it is that is afraid of public scrutiny.[11]

As Rand Paul astutely pointed out, "If all-encompassing government requires all-encompassing force, perhaps pervasive government's 'success' is proportional to the willingness of its leaders to use force."[12] If you want a government that can control every little facet of peoples' lives – when they can leave their house, how far they can travel from their home, whether or not they can work, if they can visit family, if they can hug somebody, if they can show their face in public – the only way that you'll be successful in your policies is if you have wicked men who are more than willing to follow orders.

One Flew Over the Cuckoo's Nest

In what is possibly one of the most terrifying scenes of the novel *One Flew Over the Cuckoo's Nest*, a group of psychiatry students examine the inmates of an asylum one-by-one. One of the residents being examined is perfectly sane, yet despite this, the students are able to "diagnose" him with a *number* of mental disorders. The same can easily be done with public health, and once an issue becomes politicized, using psychological "disorders" to brand those who believe differently than one's self is the beginning of the dehumanization of others and the subsequent avalanche of acts of terror that will follow.

When Brazilian researchers "discover" that those who shun face masks are more likely to be sociopaths, and to exhibit traits such as narcissism, Machiavellianism, and psychopathy – the dark triad of personality traits – should one accepts such research at face value, or should one realize that politicization of an issue quickly leads to biased "science"?[13]

What does such "science" set the stage for, if not the ability to perform inhuman acts against those who are no longer viewed as human? Does this set the stage for political opponents being branded as having a dangerous mental disorder? And then what? Reeducation? Asylums? Forced medication? Execution? There is nothing new under the sun, and such has most certainly happened before. Why believe that the above is a stretch of the imagination?

Keep in mind that these were the exact same types of studies that came out of Germany for years in the 1930s detailing how the Jewish race was anything but human. How they were a race of inbreds, genetically unfit to associate with the rest of humanity. You already know the consequences of such a philosophy. Have we seen the same within the US? Have we seen the same type of philosophy take place in modern times?

Well, it is *because* of such logic that couples without face masks are hauled off of New York City ferries by the NYPD to the cheers of a nearby crowd. In the beginning of September 2020, the captain of a ferry ordered a couple to put on face masks. They refused, stating that they were exempt from the April 17 executive order because they suffered from medical conditions that prevented them from wearing face masks. When the cops showed up, they then asked to see proof of the medical condition. The couple then got a summons for disorderly conduct, as a cop at the scene referred to the couple as knuckleheads.[14]

Let's examine this. To begin with, medical information is private and no cop has any right or authority to ask for proof of a medical condition. Secondly, is the forced masking of someone with a medical condition truly an act of virtue to the point that it deserves applause as those who can't mask are hauled away in chains? This should come as Exhibit A for those who believe that there aren't police officers, public health officials, or even members of the public who won't readily violate others' human rights should they feel like it.

Once an issue becomes politicized, people will go to drastic resorts to push through what they believe is the proper political approach. It no longer matters what actual morality states. Once you've successfully robbed another person of their humanity, you have mentally freed yourself from feeling any form of guilt for whatever actions you take against them. After all, if you mentally believe that they are vermin, why should your actions reflect any differently? You'll go around *looking* for reasons to lock people up.

Take Montgomery County, Maryland, for example. It was there that Travis Gayles, a county health officer, announced there would be a $5000 fine *and up to a year in prison* punishment for private school teachers who taught students in person between August 8, 2020, to October 1. His justification for such an action was that there had been an increase in COVID cases in DC, Virginia, and other regions of Maryland. At the time, however, Montgomery County COVID cases were at incredibly low levels (actually 0.000008% of the populace, if my math is correct). Later, Governor Larry Hogan overruled Gayles' decree, saying that it was too broad of a rule and inconsistent with the powers that are delegated to his office. Hogan stated, "This is a decision for schools and parents, not politicians."

Gayle responded two days later by issuing a further decree that local health officers were entitled to "take any action or measure necessary to prevent the spread of communicable disease." According to Gayles, as long as there were 8 positive tests each day in Montgomery County, he had the right to shut down all private schools until at least October 1. "The purpose of what we're doing is to keep kids safe," Gayles added.[15] The Constitution, the protection of human rights no longer matters to people who have deemed others to be unsafe. They'll do whatever they want to accomplish whatever they want. To be sure, their actions will be explained away, but that by no means means they'll be justified.

Atilis Gym

One of the most exciting aspects of 2020 was watching the story of Atilis Gym unfold. The Bellmawr, New Jersey gym was owned by true patriots who refused to cave to the unlawful demands of local health authorities. Despite not having a single case of COVID being traced back to his gym, the owner of Atilis Gym was *forced* to close by the government. The gym was seeing 500-700 visitors on a daily basis. If 500-700 people are willing to "take the risk" to go to their gym during a "pandemic", why must they be forbidden from doing so? Their actions don't hurt anybody else, so what is the real issue here?

The owner of Atilis Gym was being fined $15,497.76 every day that he stayed open, and up until December 10, 2020, he had received over *60* citations, coming to an amount of $1.2 million in fines. Keep in mind he was being fined by health authorities who had zero evidence that his gym was the cause of anybody being sick, and was being fined for *going to work*.[16]

Ian Smith, 33, and Frank Trumbetti, 51, the two owners of Atilis Gym were harassed throughout the entire COVID panic. They were arrested on charges of contempt of court after refusing to comply with a judge ordered shutdown of their gym in late July 2020, charged with violating a disaster control act, and with obstruction as well.[17] Just days after they were released from jail, they arrived to work to find that the government had installed *barriers* to *their* gym. In response, they kicked through the barriers and reopened.

Smith had this to say: "Governor Murphy has weaponized the police force against us over and over. I think he looks foolish, the way he's treating us – he's pulling out all the stops. You have to ask, how far will one man go to destroy a small business?"

As of early August 2020, officials were considering revoking the gym's business license, forcing the gym to shut down permanently. This, despite the owners having already limited their gym's capacity to 25%, monitoring client temperatures upon entering, asking members to sign specialized COVID waivers, giving each member their own disinfectant spray, and installing a new air purification system within the gym.[18]

To further add fuel to the fire was a December 2020 study performed in Colorado by the International Health, Racquet, and Sports Club Association that found that gym attendance has *not* been linked to any outbreaks within that state. The study collected data from 49 million gym check ins, finding that there were only 1155 cases that could be possibly linked to gym attendance. In other words, 0.0023% of gym check-ins ended up sick. The Oregon Consulting

Group was then brought on to analyze the findings in order to further prove that the data was accurate and not a misrepresentation.[19]

This is what I'm talking about. When governments are given unlimited authority – or when they take what is not theirs, when they reach across the bounds to act where they have no legal ability to do so – and the people do nothing to stop it, then you will end up with tyranny every single time. You will end up with men and women being locked up for simply going to their jobs. For attempting to be able to feed themselves, pay their medical bills, send their kids to school, and so on. And often, when only a few are brave enough to fight for what is right, it is not enough.

Little Pig, Little Pig, Let Us In

The year 2020 saw further extremes taken by law enforcement than we had ever seen before. It was in late October 2020 that UK law enforcement announced that they were going to enter peoples' homes and break up Christmas gatherings if the occupants were found in violation of COVID regulations. The West Midland police and crime commissioner David Jamieson announced, "It's not the police's job to stop people enjoying their Christmas, however, we are there to enforce the rules that the government makes, and if the government makes those rules, then the government has to explain that to the public.[20]

In other words, "I'm just doing my job, ma'am. Now get in the train."

Jamieson appears to have forgotten that he *is* part of the government, and instead has chosen to deflect the blame (his own) onto somebody else. Most certainly a government will make laws, but that by no means automatically indicates that all of them are just or should be followed. A government stamp of approval on a particular piece of legislation does not equal morality. If such were the case, then we seriously could not find fault with any of the Nazi soldiers who shipped Jews to Auschwitz. They were just following orders, after all. And the secret police of Hitler were as well. They were simply automatons, programmed to do one particular thing – obey and enforce the government's every whim without once even *thinking*. It's a result of this level of stupidity, cowardice, and blatant disrespect of other human beings that tyranny is able to flourish throughout the world.

As Frederic Bastiat pointed out in his book *The Law*, law does not equal justice.[21] Just because something has been etched into the lawbooks of a society does *not* mean that it is necessarily morally right. Examine the forced child sacrifice of the Incan empire, where a third of all 13-year-old girls were ritually murdered.[22] Examine the presence of slavery throughout world history. Consider the "legalization" of forced prostitution in some societies. For further proof of such, analyze this conversation between Tuvia Bielski, a Jewish partisan during World War 2, and a Belorussian man who had turned over 18 Jews – men, women, and children – to the slaughterhouse of the Nazi system:

"How can a man with a conscience turn over people that will be killed? Why are you doing this?"

"What do you mean, sir? It is the law. We have to obey the law."[23]

The point is that law does not necessarily equal justice. Too many minds have become blinded to this very simple truth. They believe that simply because a judge, congressman, or health authority has issued some edict, that it of necessity is righteous to follow. Consider these past examples from history – consider the current institutes of wickedness you see legalized within our current society – and ask yourself this question: do you believe the same?

9

"The Laws Are For Thee, Not For We."

*"What an affront to the King of the universe, to maintain
that the happiness of a monster sunk in debauchery and
spreading desolation and murder among men, of a
Caligula, a Nero, or a Charles, is more precious in His
sight than that of millions of His suppliant creatures, who
do justice, love mercy, and walk humbly with their God!"*
– Samuel Adams[1]

The Founding Fathers of America understood that all men
are created equal. Nobody is better than another simply for
the fact that he was born. Our entire Constitution and Bill of
Rights was built with the understanding that all men's being
created equal was a foundational pillar of what it means to
live in America. And this is truly a beautiful understanding.
It is such an understanding that places Americans on an
equal footing with each other in regard to the law.

This is not to say that some may not be borne in more
advantageous positions than another – the man who is born
into a well-established and wealthy family is going to likely
have an easier go of life than the man who is born into an
orphanage with nothing. But that is not the point. The *point*
is that in the eyes of American law – which was originally
written with a very clear understanding of mankind's God-
given rights – both of these men are absolutely equal.

One does not get better or preferable treatment over the other simply because of who he is. Without such a principle being a cornerstone of American law, we would quickly devolve into favoritism, nepotism, and a separation of two distinct castes of law – one for the common man, and one for the elite.

Law must be the same for everyone regardless of position in order to be truly just. Even within the span of public health, we need to ensure that law is equally applied. Yet one of the most blatant subjects which we can examine to see if this principle is being applied or not within American society is within the field of public health. Particularly with the coronavirus panic of 2020.

Instead of seeing law being applied equally, we saw the direct inverse. We saw the creation of two distinct castes within the United States: those who decree, and those who must obey.

On August 31, of 2020, Democrat Nancy Pelosi, Speaker of the House, was caught on security footage attending eSalon, a hair salon in San Francisco, at 3:08PM to get her hair washed and blow dried. Lockdowns and other draconian restrictions had long been set in place (for several months) throughout the entire US at this time, and local ordinances within San Francisco had kept salons closed since March due to the believed threat of COVID.

Erica Kious, owner of the salon, had been told that she could reopen her salon on September 1 for outdoor services only. Like most hair salons, Erica rents out her chairs to her stylists, and one of her stylists took care of Pelosi. As of the time that Pelosi received her services, Erica had already lost approximately 60% of her clientele due to the government-imposed restrictions. Erica, who is a single mother with two children, had no income throughout the entirety of the shutdown. At the time, San Francisco ordinances had made blow drying hair illegal within the city. Though *outside services* were made legal, her salon specializes in hair color, and using chemicals outside is *also* prohibited. Her business was essentially banned to the public. She had initially expected to be able to open in July, and had prepared her space for such, but then was told that she could not – despite her following all regulations that San Francisco had given her at that time.

Pelosi was caught on camera without a mask and with wet hair, which she later had blow-dried. She thus was guilty of two health code violations within San Francisco at the time. Pelosi's spokesman, Drew Hammill later said that Pelosi had indeed followed all of the rules, and that "the speaker always wears a mask and complies with local COVID requirements," despite video evidence to the contrary. San Francisco guidelines specifically state, "any service that requires your customer to remove their face covering are not permitted at this time." Nancy Pelosi then had the gall to demand that eSalon owed her an apology, stating that she had been "set up".[2,3]

Quite possibly one of the first cases of a politician violating their own rules occurred with Virginia's governor, Ralph Northam. After locking down the state of Virginia and forbidding travel, Northam was allegedly spotted at his North Carolina beach home.[4] He was also caught in late May 2020 without a face mask after declaring he'd issue a rule mandating masks outdoors.[5]

Pennsylvania witnessed similar outrages. Rachel Levine, a cross-dressing transvestite biological man who happened to be the premier *health* official of Pennsylvania ordered that COVID-positive patients be placed in nursing homes, despite their being a wealth of information at this point that

COVID could potentially be most dangerous to the frail elderly. Of the state's 3806 COVID deaths as of May of 2020, 2611 of them occurred in nursing homes and long-term care facilities. This order didn't affect him, however. Right after issuing the order, he quietly removed his *own* mother from her nursing home.[6]

Aside from being personally responsible for those deaths that were 100% related to COVID, what can be said for the message that this brings? Not only is this man not even mentally stable enough to know what gender he is, but he is in charge of the health policies of an entire state!

About two months later in Washington DC, we saw another example of the laws only applying to the little people. The Mayor of DC issued Order 2020-080, titled "Wearing of Masks in the District of Columbia to Prevent the Spread of COVID-19". This decree forced people to wear masks in businesses, apartment commons, and so on. Businesses – who had already been almost decimated by COVID-related "laws" by this point, mind you – were also told via this order that they could not patronize customers who did not wear masks, *even if both parties were ok with such*. Even while walking outdoors, people within DC were forced by this order to wear a mask *perchance* they should come within 6' of somebody.

However, there was one very interesting clause within the mayor's order that deserves a closer look. It reads as such, "The enforcement provisions of this Order shall not be applied to persons in the judicial or legislative branches of the District government while those persons are on duty; and shall not apply to any employees of the federal government while they are on duty."[7]

So in other words, *you* have to wear a mask while you're at work, while *you* are out in public, while you are walking outside, but the government doesn't have to. Why? Well, because some animals are more equal than others.

If we look at Chicago - where quite possibly the most incompetent politician within the entire US resides - we found the entire city being rocked by violent riots throughout the summer of 2020. In fact, Mayor Lightfoot seemed to encourage the riots around her city by stating that black lives are "more important than downtown corporations", particularly the downtown corporations that were being systematically looted and trashed in Chicago.

Around August 20, Mayor Lightfoot of Chicago was found to have ordered over 100 cops to guard her and her lesbian wife's home in Logan Square. People were allowed to burn Chicago to the ground everywhere else, just not in front of *her* home. It was found that as many as 140 officers were assigned to her home at certain times. In response to accusations that she was being hypocritical and giving herself special protection, Lightfoot responded that she had "a right to make sure that my home is secure," and that she had a "right in our home to live in peace." She also vehemently denied that there were hundreds of police stationed near her home. This despite their being evidence of cops being positioned outside of her home 24/7 in addition to her 24/7 personal police protection.

Lightfoot seemed to be angry when confronted with such accusations. She said, "I'm not going to make any excuses for the fact that, given the threats that I have personally received, given the threats to my home and my family, I'm going to do everything I can to make sure they're protected."

The order for large numbers of police officers to patrol her home came amidst a time when record numbers of Chicago Police Department officers were resigning and retiring due to the anti-cop climate amongst not only the liberal communities throughout the city, but within the public offices as well, where there had been a strong call to defund the police.[8,9]

This makes one wonder if she ever thought about the thousands of others throughout her city whom she left to the wolves.

Lightfoot is not the only one in Chicago who can't seem to follow her own rules, and who seems to think that they are a member of an upper caste. Chicago Alderman Tom Tunney was caught around December 7, 2020, violating both state and city coronavirus lockdown rules by allowing diners to eat at *his* restaurant. He later stated that it was indeed an "error in judgment," but attempted to justify his position by saying he only had a limited number inside, all his patrons were social distancing, and that they were wearing masks inside as well.[10]

The City Council of Minneapolis struggled with similar security-related hypocrisies. After a "veto-proof" majority of the council voted to abolish the city police department, the council then used *taxpayer provided* city funds to hire around the clock private security (via the companies Aegis and BelCom) *for themselves*. The price of such was $4500 per day, and within three weeks the council had racked up a bill of $60,000. When confronted on the issue, one of the members of the city council, Andrea Jenkins, stated that she's been pushing for her own private security detail since she was sworn in, due to Minneapolis' problems with a "large number of white nationalists."[11]

When you consider that "nationalists" is the new leftist term for "patriots", it's clear that what Jenkins *really* saw as a problem were white Americans who loved being American. This is rather ironic as well when you consider that it was Antifa and BLM who were burning Minneapolis to the ground. And I haven't forgotten the hubris behind depriving American people of protection – one of the most foundational reasons behind having a government at all – and then saying, "You know what, *we* deserve protection. This government exists to serve *us*, not the people who voted us in. Not the people we are being paid to serve." [my words, not hers].

By this point you've probably recognized that these politicians seem to always have some form of justification for why they broke their own rules. You'll notice that's a trend in report after report we have of their doing so. For instance, look at Denver's Mayor Hancock. He urged everyone before the Thanksgiving holiday to stay home and avoid any unnecessary travel. He was caught all of *30 minutes* later boarding a plane to head to Mississippi with his wife and daughter to celebrate his daughter's new job that she had taken – all in violation of his own COVID orders. His response? "I decided it would be safer for me to travel to see them than to have two family members travel back to Denver."[12]

Keep in mind that he thinks it's ok for *him* to measure the risks and make appropriate decisions, but he doesn't believe that the rest of Denver has such a capability. In fact, he pushed to make it illegal for others to do so.

Nothing Like Having the Restaurant to Yourself

Hancock isn't the only politician with a weakness for restaurants after creating COVID restrictions against them. Philadelphia's mayor, Jim Kenney, shut down his entire city, making it so that indoor dining within Philly was illegal and wasn't set to resume until September 8, and even then at only 25% capacity, on top of several other strict regulations. "We need to follow what we are being asked to do by the health department. I beg you to follow the rules," Kenney said. Later he was found eating at a friend's restaurant in Maryland without a mask. He later apologized, and then said, "Looking forward to reopening indoor dining soon and visiting my favorite spots."[13]

This is akin to putting a band-aid over a bullet hole through the heart. After you have completely demolished peoples' livelihoods, stolen their freedom, wrecked their savings, and then have the audacity to go somewhere else to eat out, you give a lame-wristed apology!? If you clearly don't believe that eating out at a restaurant is dangerous – when your own actions are proof of such – why do you behave as if such is the case in your own state? Do infectious diseases respect state boundaries?

It's not just the politicians either who are at fault here. Even doctors played along. After strongly recommending that people avoid crowds, avoid unnecessary travel, and not go out in public without a mask, Dr. Fauci was caught being one of the only people permitted into an MLB baseball game where he was photographed hanging out with two others, all three of them without masks. It's not ok for the general public to go to a baseball game, it's not ok for them to hang out at all with those they love, and it's most certainly not ok for them to do so without a mask, yet what did we find?[14] We found that apparently Dr. Fauci gets to live by different rules and recommendations than the rest of us.

Dr. Mikhail Varshavski, known as "the world's hottest doctor", repeatedly called for *mandatory* mask laws and social distancing. He was later shown photographed on a boat in Sunset Harbor surrounded by bikini-clad women - all maskless. He apparently enjoyed himself as there were photographs of his laying his head in one woman's lap as her half-naked breasts can be seen from above. But I suppose COVID can't get you when you're a doctor.[15]

Returning to the restaurant theme, November 2020 found California's governor, Gavin Newsom, having a 50th birthday party for Jason Kinney, a lobbyist and one of his top advisors, at one of California's most ritzy restaurants, The French Laundry. As of that time, California regulations limited social gatherings of any kind to members of no more than three households, and Newsom himself had dictated that people only leave their homes for "essential" purposes. After being caught after the fact, Newsom's representative did not dispute that there were more than three households present but *did* deny the party violated their own guidelines, saying that Newsom had not only done nothing wrong, but that he had "followed public health guidelines and the restaurant's protocols. Which state's guidelines they were referring to is unclear, but it was most certainly not California's. Newsom later said that he had made "an error in judgment."[16,17]

Newsom hasn't been the only hypocrite found at The French Laundry, however. San Francisco's mayor, London Breed, a Democrat, threw her own party for one of her friend's birthday party there just a few days later. Apparently, the lessons from Newsom's mistakes went unheeded.

She announced a few days after being found out that there were going to be more severe COVID restrictions on the way. One can't help but wonder whether or not this was a retributive strike? It almost appears as if she was saying, "You humiliate me? Then I will destroy you." She clearly didn't think that COVID was a big enough problem to keep her from going out, so why did she days later decree that others couldn't? Maybe she liked having the restaurant to herself?[18]

Three days after the party she also admonished people to respect social distancing, despite clearly not doing so just a matter of days before. On November 10, 2020, Breed was also found saying, "I cannot emphasize enough how important it is that everyone act responsibly to reduce the spread of the virus." So, if going out to eat and throwing birthday parties with friends has been deemed by Breed to be a responsible action, why can't anyone else do so?[19]

LA County Supervisor Sheila Kuehl also found it difficult to abide her own rules. After calling *outdoor* dining a "most dangerous situation" and voting to ban outdoor dining at restaurants, she was caught *hours* later dining outside at Il Forno Trattoria in Santa Monica.[20]

One has to begin to wonder when one reads these stories: what are these people thinking? Do they truly think that their constituents are that stupid, that they won't be watched after making a tyrannical decision that they have no authority to make in the first place?

No More Holidays

Thanksgiving and Christmas also both ended up being a source of contention among politicians and their constituents during 2020. One day before Thanksgiving, San Jose Mayor Sam Liccardo told people on Twitter that gathering for the holiday with friends and family would be dangerous. "Let's cancel the big gatherings this year and focus on keeping each other safe," he said. He then celebrated with his elderly parents at their Saratoga home with an unknown number of guests.[21]

He later apologized, saying, "I apologize for my decision to gather for Thanksgiving with my family, contrary to the rules," going on to say, "I commit to do better."[22]

Wouldn't it be wonderful if such an approach worked for the rest of us? If we could be found guilty of some tyrant's decree, and then all we had to do to get out of the consequences was sheepishly grin and lisp, "I'm sorry" as we wring our hands behind our back with our head hung low.

New York's Governor Cuomo seemed to have similar problems following his own orders. Initially on November 18, Cuomo told reporters during a conference call that his "personal advice is you don't have family gatherings – even for Thanksgiving." He also said, "This year, if you love someone, it is better and safer to stay away." Then on November 23 he had the gall to tell New Yorkers that he may host his 89-year-old mother, Matilda, for Thanksgiving.[23]

Austin, Texas mayor Steve Adler also seemed to have a problem at Thanksgiving time. While attending an outdoor wedding and reception with 20 guests for his daughter at a fancy hotel in downtown Austin, Adler told his constituents to stay home to stay safe in November. Right after this – and I do mean *right* after this – he boarded a private jet for Cabo San Lucas, Mexico – where he vacationed at his family timeshare for a week. Only one night into his relaxing Mexican vacation, Adler told his constituents back home in the United States, "We need to stay home if you can. This is not the time to relax. We are going to be looking really closely...We may have to close things down if we are not careful."

There's no time quite like family vacation time in a foreign country to be giving veiled threats to your constituents about how you may decide to ruin their lives on a whim should they decide to ignore your ideas while you do so yourself.

Adler later stated that he broke no law with his personal decisions. At the time of his daughter's wedding, the city of Austin was recommending people to avoid groups larger than ten. In an interview the first week of December, Adler said that he and his family had also poured hours of consideration into how to hold both the wedding and the vacation as safely as possible. Because you know, it's ok if he decides to measure risk and reward to make his own decisions. *You* cannot be trusted to make the same decisions, however. Adler also stated that *his* conduct was different from the other officials who were caught in hypocritical and illegal actions because *he* did not behave in a way inconsistent with his message. The man told others to stay at home and then hopped on a plane to Mexico. Tell me, is that consistent behavior?

Even judges don't seem to be immune to the temptation to violate their own laws. Judge Bill Gravell – Republican – of Williamson County, ended up violating his own stay-home-order by visiting his grandson on his birthday.[24]

To his credit, he *did* pay the $1000 fine, but judging by the lawyer's houses that I have seen in my town, that's probably a rather easy price to pay for a judge. It must be nice to be able to say, "Yeah, it's $1000 to see my grandson, but heck, *I* can afford it, so why not?" It's also unclear to me how a member of the judicial branch is able to get away with acting as if he is a part of the legislative branch of government. In American society, all three branches are separated with very distinct abilities. No branch can cross its proper bounds of authority by engaging in another branch's actions. So how did a judge create a stay-at-home order?

Even self-proclaimed president of the United States, Joe Biden wasn't immune to the idea of making laws that only applied to the little people. Just hours after mandating that people wear masks on federal property, Biden was found at the Lincoln Memorial – federal property – without a face mask. The defense given by the Queen of 'circling back', Jen Psaki, stated that it was ok that Biden didn't have a face mask on. He was outside "celebrating" his recent "win" as POTUS. As a result, he didn't need to obey the very mandate that he had made for the rest of Americans.

This was just the first of a string of executive orders – the most in American history – that Joe Biden signed. And he violated it himself within the span of a few short hours.[25]

So when it comes to public health, is it too much to ask that those who make the policy and laws regarding such follow their own rules? Law should equally apply to all, not just to the peons of society. For without such, that' exactly what happens: a large percentage of a nation are transformed against their will into nothing other than peons.

Unequal Laws

Another interesting facet of unequal treatment under the law that we saw throughout 2020 was in the way that public health was utilized as a weapon against those who went against the political status quo. In short, this was a different example of hypocrisy.

One of the more heartbreaking scenes demonstrating such came in December 2020 from LA restaurant owner Angela Marsden. Angela owned the Pineapple Hill Saloon and Grill in Sherman Oaks. Due to LA banning outdoor dining in November, she was told that she could no longer legally serve customers outside. This came after Angela had spent approximately $80,000 making her restaurant compliant with the most recent string of COVID regulations for restaurants. She posted a video on social media demonstrating the hypocrisy taking place just *feet* away from her, however.

It was a mere couple of feet from her restaurant that a Hollywood crew had set up an outdoor dining area that looked virtually the same as what she had set up at the Pineapple Hill Saloon. Yet hers was deemed to be dangerous and illegal, while Hollywood was enabled to continue on with the exact same set up.[26]

What reasoning can be given for allowing those within the realm of the media to continue on, while individuals – the common man – is not allowed to have a business to provide for oneself and family? Marsden's restaurant had been open for 40 years by this point. Yet due to unequal treatment under the law, she said that there was a very real threat she may have to close down permanently by February 2021. The only reason that comes to this author's mind as to why this discrepancy exists is because one citizen can serve as a source of propaganda, while the other cannot.

A similar case occurred on Staten Island during the same month. Daniel Presti, the co-owner of a bar called Mac's, had his liquor license pulled due to lockdown violations. Seeing that numerous locations throughout the country had declared themselves "autonomous zones" and left to be by government authorities, Presti decided to do the same, declaring his bar an autonomous zone. Not only would this theoretically allow him to remain open and create his own law – as it had throughout much of the rest of the country – but his no longer selling drinks, instead *giving* them away and taking donations was a loophole in the current law as well.

Plainclothes cops had been watching Presti, however, and when they spotted 14 people eating and drinking – despite the ban – within the bar, they moved in and arrested Presti. He was in turn charged with obstructing governmental administration and continuing to operate a business despite being in an "orange zone" where indoor dining wasn't allowed and there was a 10PM curfew.[27]

This came at a time when big department store style businesses were allowed to stay open. Yet, small business owners throughout the country were not.

None of this is an example of a just society.

Proper law is equally applied to all citizens throughout a society, regardless of creed, political views, education, background or office. This is the only way to have a truly free and truly just society. Anything else only breeds corruption and causes people to realize that the only way that they can truly be protected from the law is to do what they can to get above it.

As Samuel Adams said in his excellent essay "The Rights of the Colonists as Men", "There should be one rule of justice for rich and poor, for the favorite at court, and the countryman at the plough."[28] Other early American patriots understood the same to be the case. Thomas Paine famously wrote that "...in America THE LAW IS KING."[29]

Within the United States, it is the Constitution that is the supreme law of the land, and nothing within it states that there are to be separate castes of laws for separate castes of people. This is a fundamental facet of human rights. You cannot keep human rights within public health without ensuring that the laws apply equally. When a subset of society is able to issue laws for the rest of society *that do not apply to themselves*, you can be assured that tyranny is only a short duration of time away.

10

"Uhhh, We Were Wrong."

Further proof that the government should have as limited role as possible within the day-to-day lives of citizens came in droves throughout the entire COVID panic. Humans are inherently flawed creatures. Nobody on this earth is perfect, and a government worker is just as likely to be wrong as a private citizen is. However, there is something sinister about being damaged by a wrong decision made by somebody in power over you compared with being damaged by one's own wrong decision.

Consider the man who willfully chooses to not wear a seatbelt. Should he end up hitting a deer where he suffers major spine trauma, he only has himself to blame. Now – for the sake of argument – consider a government that has decided that seat belts are dangerous, and therefore, they've made it illegal for people to use them. The government has robbed individuals of their ability to make their own decisions. People have been robbed of their freedom to choose.

In such a case, if a man hit a deer and suffered major spine trauma, he would know that the sole cause of such was due to the government's decisions. Others in positions of power above him decided that they could choose but he could not, and he suffered as a result. This adds a tremendous amount of pain to any already existing injury. While this is most certainly a rather silly analogy, the point remains: when somebody is injured as a direct result of following government policy in an arena where government should not have been involved in the first place, injustice has taken place.

It's a result of this – a result of this respect for human freedom as well as an understanding of man's own fallibility – that public health workers need to let freedom reign throughout the field of public health. All too often, public health workers are wrong, and the end result is people being injured against their will. As usual, there are some fantastic examples of such that we can glean from the 2020 COVID panic.

Intervening with Medicine

In the initial stages of the COVID situation it was found that hydroxychloroquine (HCQ) may show some promise in treating those who were infected with the virus. This would have been a fine and acceptable form of treatment, but the problem came when President Trump announced that HCQ may be a valid form of treatment. In unison, the entire mainstream media turned against HCQ with a vengeance. Study after study was *crafted* proving that HCQ was dangerous, had no benefits, and would lead to a false sense of security among those who were infected with COVID.

Doctors were actually banned from prescribing HCQ – a medicine that they had been permitted to prescribe just days prior – by both hospitals and medical groups throughout the country. The decision to treat the patient in a way that a doctor found to be both safe and effective was removed from the doctor.[1]

The Lancet, a once prominent and leading medical journal, actually published a study "proving" that hydroxychloroquine was not only ineffective in COVID patients, but actually increased their risk of death as well. It was a direct result of this study – this provision of further ammo against Trump – that *nations* banned HCQ for being a valid form of COVID treatment. The problem came upon further inspection of the study, however. Over 100 scientists and clinicians questioned the study results, and upon further inspection, it was found that the study had utilized shoddy data to formulate its results.

The study had actually utilized a massive hospital database owned by Chicago company Surgisphere. Red flags were raised when it was found that Surgisphere's data didn't actually line up with what the government was reporting. It turned out that Surgisphere appears to be a sham company. As of June 3, 2020, there were only three employees reported as working at Surgisphere – all of whom had little to no data or scientific work background. In fact, one of the employees – listed as a marketing executive – was an adult model and events hostess. I'm not sure how she was "marketing" Surgisphere. Another employee – listed as a science editor – appeared to be a fantasy artist and science fiction writer. When the company website was examined, it was found that the "get in touch" link on the homepage redirected to a Wordpress template for a cryptocurrency website. This was quickly changed afterwards.

Because of all this, *The Lancet* was forced to issue a statement – an apology of sorts - on June 2, 2020.[2] However, the damage had already been done. States had made their decisions, and they were sticking to their guns. Instead of HCQ, a newer medication was now recommended for those diagnosed with COVID – Remdesivir.

This drug was widely lauded as a fantastic treatment for COVID, and hospitals throughout America began to use it to treat their patients. However, by October of 2020, a study showed that Remdesivir was found to have no substantial effect on a COVID patient's chances of survival. To be fair, this study also found HCQ to be ineffective in combating COVID, but the point remains that people were being treated with something that was later found to be ineffective.[3] It was only a month later that the World Health Organization officially recommended that doctors shouldn't prescribe Remdesivir to their patients.[4]

The main point that I would like to discuss with this though is the use of politics to refuse a valid medical treatment to a patient. While this particular study found

HCQ to be ineffective in treating patients, it wasn't that study that resulted in the medicine being banned or refused to be filled by pharmacies throughout the US. Instead, it was politics and propaganda that did so. Because one man suggested this as a potential remedy it had to be opposed at all costs and anybody who would even go so far as to think that HCQ was a valid form of treatment therefore deserved to be criticized endlessly and silenced. As mentioned, some doctors even had the threat of losing their medical license hang over their heads by authorities who had now deemed themselves responsible for controlling what a doctor could prescribe for a patient.

Public health authorities should never intervene in such unless there is a clear and present danger from such taking place. If we end up in a situation where we find that a medication is clearly causing birth defects in the children of mothers who have been given the medicine – such as with thalidomide – then absolutely, something must be done. However, if we're talking about a drug with over 70 years of research behind it, that's been proven safe, why are we refusing to let both a doctor and a patient come to an agreement regarding how things are going to proceed treatment-wise?

Oops.

The year of 2020 saw more gargantuan public health decisions on a worldwide scale than has ever happened before in history. Though the Black Death and the Spanish Flu affected much of the world as well, the government response to both of those pandemics came nowhere near the scope of what the world saw with COVID. As the reader has probably already discovered by this point, much of those decisions – potentially even most of them – were terrible.

Asides from violating human rights and the American Constitution, a great many of them had rather severe side effects and consequences those involved in the public health sector were either incapable of seeing due to incompetence (*not* because the end results were actually impossible to foresee) or due to sheer evil.

Depression and Suicide

Prime among these examples would be the toll on mental health that came about as a *direct result* of public health authorities' decisions. A November 12, 2020, CDC report suggested that COVID and the response to it was taking a devastating toll on the mental health of children. The average weekly numbers of children's visits to emergency departments for mental health reasons had absolutely soared by this point. Compared with 2019, the number of visits to the ER for children aged 5 – 11 had increased by 24%, and the number of visits to ERs for mental health issues among kids aged 12 – 17 had increased by 31%.

According to the report, "Many mental disorders commence in childhood, and mental health concerns in these age groups might be exacerbated by stress related to the pandemic and abrupt disruptions to daily life associated with mitigation efforts, including anxiety about illness, social isolation, and interrupted connectedness to school."[5]

The implications of such are concerning. This means that not only were children mentally scarred from The Panic during 2020 after being forcibly separated from all of their friends and family, but that there are going to potentially be lifelong consequences for these children. Many of them are likely to now develop permanent mental illnesses and disorders that will haunt them (and those they love) for the rest of their lives.

And such didn't have to be.

It didn't have to turn out that way, and yet it did. Children didn't have to have their minds marred, and yet it happened. All because of the decisions made by mainstream media, public health authorities, and politicians. However, even parents are to blame in many of these cases. Some parents posted stories on Twitter about how the most difficult part about the pandemic was having to listen to their 5-year-old cry and ask to be let out after the parent *locked them in their room alone for two weeks.* And why was this? Because the child was allegedly exposed to someone at their school.[6]

There is no sugar coating here. This is child abuse. There is no justification for such an action by a parent to their child not far removed from diapers during a global misinformation war. Will that child grow up normal, or will that child grow up with devastating memories etched into his psyche for the rest of his earthly life? You tell me.

Children weren't the only ones who struggled with mental health throughout 2020. According to a study published in JAMA Network, as of mid-April of 2020 the prevalence of depression within the US was more than three-fold higher compared with the most recent population-based estimates of mental health.[7] For California it was even worse. They actually experienced a *year's* worth of suicides within the span of *one month.*[8]

But can we be surprised that this actually happened? During this point of time there was still a massive amount of fear and uncertainty floating through the air. Nobody really knew what was going on or what the extent of the damage was going to be. All anybody really knew was that something scary had come out of China, that China had engaged in the largest quarantine in history, and that whatever it was that China was scared about was popping up throughout the rest of the world.

When you combine this with the wave of lockdowns, of unemployment, of social isolation, and other policy-driven decisions that were floating around out there, it almost *has* to be expected that there are going to be increased rates of depression. Why did other states not see that many suicides though? Why just California? I would argue that the catalyst was government response. California was widely noted for having some of the most severe COVID regulations throughout all of America – people were essentially stripped of all of their freedoms overnight. So yes, while fear most certainly played a factor in things, I believe that government policy was what in fact pushed many people over the edge who would otherwise have made it through a turbulent time in their life.

What else did we see though? What other ripples were caused by the splash of public health officials throughout the world jumping into the water? Were there other strange and dangerous side-effects as a result of overzealousness? Yep, it sure does appear that way.

Mask Mouth

For starters, we must look no further than at the smile coming from across the room. It was August of 2020 when dentists began to come to the forefront of the discussion in certain public health circles. After the WHO began telling people to put off seeing their dentist – this due to an alleged increased risk of catching COVID-19 from being in such close proximity to somebody else for so long – many people actually ended up listening to the advice, shunning their mouths in the process.

The end result? Skyrocketing rates of gum inflammation. This came about not only from people not going to the dentist for their regular checkups, but due to other public health policies being put into place as well. Namely, mandatory masking.

Dr. Rob Ramondl, dentist and cofounder of One Manhattan Dental had this to say, "We're seeing inflammation in peoples' gums that have been healthy forever, and cavities in people who have never had them before." He went on to say that "about 50% of our patients are being impacted by this, [so] we decided to name it 'mask mouth'." Dr. Marc Sclafani, cofounder of One Manhattan Dental, added "Gum disease – or periodontal disease – will eventually lead to strokes and an increased risk of heart attacks."[9]

It's rather odd when public health officials are directly responsible for damaging the health – or even jeopardizing the lives – of the very people they publicly acclaim to care so much about, is it not? When you tell people to not see their healthcare providers, there are very easy to foresee conclusions. For further example, consider the significant drop in cancer diagnoses, heart attacks, and other chronic and potentially terminal diseases throughout 2020. It's statistically impossible for this drop to come about as a result of one year's actions. In other words, it's not a true drop.

What this drop means is that people weren't going to their doctors that should have been. People weren't getting health issues checked out, meaning that tumors had more time to grow. More chance of becoming malignant. Arteries had a further chance to clog. The end result of such is increased death and disease. And again, much of this never had to happen. It was a direct consequence of failed government policy – of governments overreaching their natural and just jurisdictions. And anytime a government does such, increased misery and death is *always* the end result.

Vaccine Issues

There were a wide number of dangers with the COVID shots that came out during The Panic. Many were rightfully concerned with injecting themselves with a concoction that had not only not received more than a year of testing (within the US, vaccines require ten years of research before they are approved for use by the FDA), but in which vaccine manufacturers had been granted full legal immunity from ill effects as well.

Despite such, governments throughout the world pushed the shot on their citizens. Was such the right decision? Is such the right decision?

In January of 2021, health experts out of Wuhan, China told other countries that they ought to suspend the use of mRNA-based COVID shots, especially among the elderly. An anonymous Beijing immunologist further recommended that no one over the age of 80 should be given such a shot. This was shortly after Norway gave 33,000 shots and had 23 people die just a short time after receiving those shots. Upon autopsy, 13 of those deaths were found to have been the result of common side effects leading to severe reactions in the frail.[10]

The COVID shot was released within the US in December/January of 2020/2021. Within the first three months, miscarriages spiked 366%. It was also found that within the same time span more people had died of COVID shots than had died from vaccines over the past 20 years combined.

Other reports showed people becoming magnetic after receiving the shot, emitting EMF radiation (typically only associated with electronics), and other anecdotal reports of people emitting Bluetooth signals after getting their COVID shot.[11]

Famine

It was in November of 2020 that the United Nations World Food Program (UNWFP) warned there was going to be a devastating famine that would likely sweep across the globe throughout 2021. The head of the UNWFP, David Beasley, went so far as to say that we were going to see "famines of Biblical proportions." This was a direct result of government-imposed lockdowns. While developed countries most certainly saw their fare share of economic destruction as a result of such policies, underdeveloped countries ended up with mass death.

In nations where large amounts of the people are engaged in a subsistence lifestyle, the lack of just one paycheck can spell disaster. Months of such left millions throughout the world starving.[12]

What Conclusions Can We Reach From Such?

The lesson to be gleaned by students of public health is this: do not assume your own infallibility. When you support regulations or laws that invade on others human liberty, you are doing just that – assuming that you are better able to make other peoples' decisions *for* them. As you can see from the above examples, infallibility is not a human trait, and it is best to let people make their own decisions.

Otherwise, you are indeed the cause for any pain that comes about as the result of the policies that you support.

11

"Well, This Will Work."

There are some decisions that people within the sphere of public health have made that make you realize stupidity can truly be found anywhere. People are promoted to their level of inability, and nowhere is this more visible than within public health. Perhaps it is because of a lack of competition that the losers are able to rise so high within this realm. Such is common throughout government office.

Or perhaps there is a darker, underlying purpose. I'll let you draw your own conclusions on such.

To illustrate stupidity though, let's say you live on a small island filled with thousands of people. Would it not be foolish to close down all of the 911 dispatch centers that you have on the island?

You may readily agree, but in fact, this is what Puerto Rico did in 2020. The entire island only has two 911 dispatching centers that field emergency calls for help. Because some of the employees at those centers tested positive for COVID, however, they were *both* shut down.

Imagine if you will what would happen if the same thing were done with hospitals. A surgeon gets COVID, and so the entire hospital is shut down, permitting no more patients. In essence, this decision shut down the police department of the island as well. How do the police know where to go if they can't be reached? Puerto Rican authorities brought a government solution to this problem by telling residents to instead dial a ten-digit phone number to reach help.[1]

How exactly would this play out?

"Help! He broke his leg!"

"Quick! Call the ambulance! What's the number?"

"It's 437-348...uhhh...is it 6 next?"

Do you see how this goes? The reason that 911 is what it is, is because it is short and easy to remember.

What about the releasing of prisoners? Does this seem like a valid way to deal with what has been coined a public health crisis? Does releasing prisoners upon the public at large truly protect the public health? One can easily see that it does not, but what one needs to understand is that such was done to not protect the public, but instead to protect the *prisoners.*

In July 2020, California announced that it plans to release 8000 inmates in order *to slow the spread of COVID.* I suppose the thought process is that if the prisoners are willing to kill others, perhaps they'll kill COVID too? It was on July 10, that the Department of Corrections and Rehabilitation announced that they were going to release prisoners in order to create more space in the prisons. As 2020 went on, it became clear that this space was to be used for business owners and political opponents.

By July of 2020, since mid-March approximately 10,000 inmates had already been released in California.[2]

Seriously. How does one expect the releasing of prisoners to affect the incidence of COVID? This author believes that the purpose of such an action is of darker design. If you want to push for stronger gun control, you need to create more incidences where people are killed. Never waste a tragedy, as the leftist saying goes, and if you release prisoners upon the public, you are bound to have more tragedies in the very near future. This then gives you the political excuse to begin to again push for stronger gun control legislation. Perhaps it's nothing more than a theory, but I truly see no other logic behind such a decision.

Are there other similar examples we can find that seem to show evidence of no thought being used whatsoever? But of course!

During December 2020, the CDC began to ask people to wear a mask whenever they were indoors, with the exception of being in one's own home. It didn't matter whether you were in a secluded office, warehouse, or wherever. If you were indoors, the CDC wanted you to wear a mask.

According to such a guideline, anytime that you would visit friends or relatives you should also wear a mask.[3]

Los Angeles mayor Eric Garcetti took things even further in December 2020. He made it so that all "unnecessary travel on foot" was banned. According to his mandate, "all travel, including, without limitation, travel on foot, bicycle, scooter, motorcycle, automobile, or public transit" was to stop in addition to the closure of all non-essential businesses.

News agencies were exempted from such an order within LA of course, and once more, I'll leave you the reader to deduce what the potential reasons for such could be.[4] Why is it unsafe for the entire city of LA to go about their daily business, but it's perfectly safe for the newsmen?

What Can We Learn From Such Behavior?

Though it should go without saying, those in positions of power in the field of public health should engage in policies that do not look as if they are throwing crap at a wall and waiting to see what sticks. Policies should show clear evidence of logic, clear concern for human rights, and be filled with common sense.

It's when policies are devoid of all three of these factors that the public at large grows distrustful against public health policy and will take steps to avoid such or resort to outright resistance altogether.

12

When Public Health is No Longer About Public Health

One of the first things that I realized throughout grad school was that there was a tendency amongst textbook writers, scientists, and policy makers to drastically expand the concept of "public health" well beyond what the term public health actually refers to.

The term quickly became something of a Swiss army knife that could be used for literally *any* topic out there; things just needed to be worded correctly. I grew rather disgusted with the misappropriation of the term. Public health refers to the things that truly involve the health of individuals. There are four main categories where I've seen the concept of public health be stretched so thin that there is no question that what is really being done is the transformation of public health into a weapon.

Racism

Throughout 2020 we witnessed the diatribe against white people turn to the extreme. BLM marched through streets burning and looting white-owned businesses and homes, while beating white people to a pulp throughout the states for no other reason than their skin color. All in the name of fighting against racism. Whites are currently the biggest victim of institutional racism throughout the United States. Through the presence of (taxpayer funded) schools' and businesses' "diversity committees" meritocracies are shattered and whites are refused entry or hire for no other reason than the color of their skin. College scholarships routinely are granted to those who are not white simply because of the color of their skin as well.

We saw further institutionalized racism throughout 2020 come in the name of public health. In December of 2020, Cornell University, what some consider a rather prestigious university, decreed that all new students must get the flu vaccine in order to attend the school. The exception to the rule was if one was black, indigenous, or a person of color.[1]

So basically, only *white* people have to get the flu shot in order to attend Cornell University from now on. Only *white* people have to have their rights and bodies violated in order to attend classes, supposedly from the reasoning that whites are harbingers of disease into a community? The scary thing about this is that it was this same line of reasoning that was tossed around 1930s Germany about Jews before the Holocaust began not long afterwards.

Lincoln County, Oregon, actually institutionalized racism within their *community*. Health officials there in June of 2020 made masks mandatory for whites while simultaneously exempting "people of color." Why? Because masks promote racial profiling of colored people, they say. According to ReNika Moore of the ACLU's Racial Justice Program, "For many black people, deciding whether or not to wear a bandana in public to protect themselves and others from contracting coronavirus is a lose-lose situation that can result in life-threatening consequences either way."[2]

Ignore the fact that a bandana isn't going to protect anybody from anything. Ignore the fact that ReNika apparently believes that black people are simply gunned down in the streets simply for being black. (To prove the *actual* situation try being a white person walking through a black neighborhood late at night. Try being a white person walking through particular parts of Hawaii late at night. While there are regions of the country where a white person *can* and *will* be gunned down solely because of their skin color, the opposite does not happen.)

Such a statement is to say that cops are automatically looking for black people to gun down. It is to say that whites are privileged. Can a white person not be afraid of police harassment? Why can a black person have the legal ability to show his face in public while a white person cannot? How is *this* not racism?

Minneapolis' City Council thought things were so bad in their area (and in reality, they were, just not in the way that the council pretended) that they declared racism a public emergency on July 17, 2020. I'm not really sure what they thought was happening there – were black people mysteriously being lynched throughout the city overnight? Was the KKK demonstrating and taking over neighborhoods? – but that is what happened. According to the council's resolution, "Racism in all its forms causes persistent discrimination and disparate outcomes in many areas of life, including housing, education, health, employment, public safety, and criminal justice; exacerbated further by the COVID-19 pandemic crisis."

What's not exactly clear to me is what they mean. Is COVID-19 a racist virus, systematically floating throughout towns at night purposefully infecting those who it deems un-white? Or is the council accusing the healthcare workers throughout their city of not treating blacks in the manner that they should be treated when they present COVID symptoms? As a healthcare worker, I would be rather angry at such an accusation leveled towards myself.

Minneapolis promised to prioritize racial equity as a result of their "crisis". The mayor's budget there was also directed towards the housing, community-based infrastructure, and small business development of those deemed to be black, indigenous, or people of color (BIPOC). So it no longer mattered if you paid a lot of taxes in your neighborhood and would like to see the streets kept up, the streetlights working, and get that necessary roundabout finally put in. Your money was going to BIPOC regions instead. Is this not redistribution of wealth? Would this not be akin to the US giving American taxpayer money to Kenya?

The council's report goes on, "A multitude of studies connect racism to inequitable health outcomes for black, indigenous, and people of color, including cancer, coronary heart disease, diabetes, hypertension, high infant and maternal mortality rates, demonstrating that racism is the root cause of social determinants of health."

What the council doesn't seem to understand (or rather is willfully ignoring to further their agenda) is that they are confusing *race* with racism. Though I don't believe that genes are destiny, there's no doubt that they most certainly have a role to play in health. For example, sickle cell primarily affects black people. That's not because sickle cell is a racist condition, a racism-caused condition, or because healthcare providers give the condition or refuse to treat the condition in those that have it. It is simply a condition that one is more prone to suffer from should one be black.

The council also seems to ignore the fact that both culture and personal choice have a lot to say about individual health as well. If your culture primarily eats unhealthy foods, then there is a greater chance that your culture will suffer from negative health outcomes. I don't believe that one can argue that this is due to racism-caused "food deserts" either, where there are no traditional grocery stores within miles of particular urban areas.

If there is no grocery store within a particular area, there are reasons for it that have nothing to do with race. Nobody will deny that there are unsafe neighborhoods and streets in their town. It's a fact of life. As an investor, would you consider investing a substantial portion of your funds into an area that you believe is dangerous? There are neighborhoods in my town that I would either be shot or beat to the point of death simply for being caught walking in them for no other reason than the color of my skin. Does that sound like the kind of place where I would be willing to set up shop? If your answer to that question is 'no' as well, then I believe we have something of an understanding when we question the concept of a "food desert" existing at all.

Burlington, Vermont was another city that stated that racism was a public health emergency. I'm not entirely sure how, seeing that Vermont has a very low percentage – just 1% of Vermont's total population - of black people who live in it, but Mayor Miro Weinberger felt the need to say, "Racism is a public health crisis. As a result of deeply embedded structural racism, black and brown Americans experience far worse outcomes than their white contemporaries." Miro went on to acknowledge that Vermont had only 1% of their population being black, but that "as of July 8th, they account for 10% of the total confirmed COVID-19 cases in Vermont." As such, Burlington has committed itself to eliminate "race-based health".[3]

Once more, Miro as well doesn't seem to understand some of the very basic tenants of health. It's not racism that creates health conditions, it's genetics and culture. Communists have never been much for the facts though.

Unsurprisingly, even New York City got in on the madness. Mayor de Blasio said on July 9, 2020 while on CNN with Wolf Blitzer that he was banning all large public gatherings within the city in order to stop COVID. Of course, the exception was made for Black Lives Matter protests.[4]

Because viruses don't attack people when they're gathering in the name of Marxism.

Personal Vendettas

Lord Acton noted that absolute power corrupts absolutely, and who in a position of power hasn't suffered from the temptation to use such to strike down those who have offended them? One of the most blatant examples of such can be found in the story of Atilis Gym, a fitness facility in New Jersey. Governor Phil Murphy put the entire state into lockdown over COVID-created fears.

The owners of Atilis refused to comply with Murphy's orders, and rightfully so. Murphy had not the authority to even put such an order into practice. The owners of Atilis Gym kept their gym open despite the lockdown orders and numerous visits from government authorities, and on August 11 had their business license revoked after the Bellmawr Borough Council voted 5-1 in favor of pulling their license.

Requiring a license to earn a living is government overreach as it is, but to threaten fines and the removal of one's ability to earn a living simply because they have the balls to stand up against tyrannical and unconstitutional decrees is absurd. The council presented *zero* evidence at their meeting that Atilis Gym posed a health risk to the community, and also refused to hold off the vote until they actually *could* present evidence that Atiliis Gym was a health risk. Furthermore, the New Jersey attorney general office recommended that there be daily fines instituted against Smith and Trumbetti to the amount of $10,000 *per day* as well as imprisonment in order to "coerce" them to comply with Phil Murphy's decree.[5]

Keep in mind that throughout this time mega corporations were still permitted to stay open and government workers were still allowed to work and earn a paycheck as well.

Politics

It's rather depressing to see politics being used as a weapon against people to infringe on basic human rights. Such is history, however, and I suppose one shouldn't be that shocked to discover career politicians are often corrupt and liars, but it still leaves one wishing for a world where such wasn't the case.

In many cases throughout 2020, we saw instances where public health wasn't ever about public health in the first place, but instead was utilized to push through a political agenda (Marxism).

For instance, New York's Governor Cuomo's office refusing to turn over COVID information to the Department of Justice. In August, the DOJ was on a fact-finding mission to determine whether the policies put in place throughout the state of New York were harmful, and if so, why they were left in place so long. Giving that the DOJ was involved, it seemed as if there was the potential for embarrassing criminal charges to be given. Typically, getting infectious disease information to somebody is a rather straightforward practice, however, in the case of Cuomo's office, they stated that they couldn't turn over the asked-for records until *two days after the presidential election of 2020* (November 5). The given reason was that the office needed more time to "find the records".

The Empire Center for Public Policy accused the New York Health Department of stalling on compliance with this Freedom of Information request for more information on the statistics involving New York's various COVID policies. Bill Hammond was the health analyst for the Empire Center who submitted the legal request. According to him, the stalling was completely unnecessary and was nothing more than a stalling tactic to avoid embarrassing Governor Cuomo, and by extension, the rest of the Democratic party as well.[6]

In short, it would be bad propaganda to have the entire Democrat party identified as the party of incompetence, corruption, theft, and death that they actually are.

Mayor Lori Lightfoot furthered her terrible image around the time of Thanksgiving by calling for residents to cancel their Thanksgiving holiday with families. This call came not even a week after she was seen amidst a large crowd celebrating the beginning stages of Joe Biden's coup. She personally issued a "Stay-at-Home" Advisory for Chicago to go in effect on November 16, saying that the people needed to "stay home unless for essential reasons" to "stop having guests over – including family members" and to "cancel traditional Thanksgiving plans".

When her hypocrisy was pointed out she responded by saying that due to peoples' being traumatized (from what is not clear), people needed time for relief. Her exact statements were, "...there are times when we actually do need to have relief and come together, and I felt like that was one of those times. That crowd was gathered whether I was there or not. But this has been a super hard year on everyone. Everyone feels traumatized."[7]

One can't help but wonder whether or not people would feel as traumatized if they didn't have a tyrant who had intruded into every aspect of their lives over the course of roughly a year.

Further evidence of public health being utilized as a political weapon occurred in November of 2020. It was during this time that New York's Governor Cuomo spoke with George Stephanopoulos of "Good Morning America" on ABC about how he had had discussions with other governors throughout the US regarding how they could collaborate a plan to block President Trump's vaccine distribution plan. Instead, Cuomo wanted to stall the vaccination plan until Joe Biden was firmly seated in the presidency.[8]

It is this author's opinion that the need for a COVID vaccine was pointless to begin with. That being said, Cuomo and the Democrat party firmly believed otherwise. If they are truly of the belief that COVID-19 is a virulent and incredibly contagious killer, would it not be sheer contempt of life to say that you *don't* want people to have access to an available vaccine in a timely manner simply because you want the credit of saving lives to go to *your* presidential candidate? There is truly no other way to look at it.

Throughout 2020 there were a number of valid talking points given that the coronavirus panic was a political stunt; the common joke being that it would disappear the day after the presidential election. Public health officials didn't do too much to discredit that popular opinion either. Los Angeles

County's Public Health Director Barbara Ferrer helped to fuel the fire when she spoke at a gathering of school nurses and other school administrators. According to Ferrer, "...we don't realistically anticipate we will be moving to tier 2 or reopening K-12 schools at least until after the election, after, you know, in early November."9

Is that not an interesting choice of words? Wouldn't it make more sense for a public health official to use some form of measurable metric to determine when schools were going to reopen? In truth, school closings don't make much scientific proof at all, but if you were going to shut down all schools, and then reopening those schools became a talking point, wouldn't it make sense to say, "We're looking at reopening schools once we are at 0.05% of our population currently being infected," or some other measurable criteria? To arbitrarily decide that school can't reopen until after a presidential election has occurred smacks of New York's Cuomo's decision that vaccine distribution needs to wait till Biden can take the credit for it, and *only* so Biden can take the credit for it.

It was also after the inauguration of Joe Biden that Washington DC began to ease restrictions on indoor dining. Likewise, after the inauguration Dr. Fauci stated that US cases were "plateauing". It was all a rather convenient timeline.10 Once Joe Biden began to live in The White House it was as if nation-wide, American governments began to relax some of the restrictions that they'd had for months. Such should raise suspicion.

The Wisconsin Department of Natural Resources played politics as well when they mandated employees wear masks *even if they're at home for virtual meetings*. The department officials stated that the purpose *wasn't* to stop infection, but instead to virtue signal that masks are important and that the Department of Natural Resources takes them seriously.[11]

Anti-Judeo-Christian Values

The attack against Judeo-Christian values has garnered momentum over the course of the last ten years, and to argue otherwise is to be politically naïve. Buddhists, Christian scientists, and wiccans are encouraged throughout the US to practice their beliefs, while Muslims in particular are routinely given special treatment – even to the point where they're allowed to marry their own brother to get them US citizenship and then allowed to hold public office. For Jews or Christians, there is a much different story, and they are routinely treated as the most hated religions within the United States (as well as the rest of the world).

This is of particular concern when you consider the fact that the United States was founded upon Judeo-Christian values, and Western civilization is built upon it. It can even be argued that there can truly be no United States without those values, for it is out of them that we get the Bill of Rights, the Declaration of Independence, and the US Constitution. If there is no Judeo-Christian foundation, there is no United States. Instead, one would quickly find themselves at the mercy of an atheistic, communist state, a caliphate, or the political chaos that is the continent of Africa.

For example of this societal attack against Christian principles, one must look no further than California – a state that likes to pretend that it has the moral high ground in being a community of love, tolerance, and widespread acceptance. That seems to be the case if you are a drug addict, transvestite, or communist there, but it by no means applies to Christians there.

Late August of 2020, Los Angeles County sent notice to famous theological author and pastor John MacArthur of Grace Community Church that they were terminating the church's parking lot lease due to the church's noncompliance with the county's lockdown restrictions. Despite the fact that the church had leased the lot from the county for *45 years*, they were told that they now had 30 days to vacate the premises or risk having their private property confiscated by the county.

The church had been open for in-person services since late July in defiance of the state's restrictions, and MacArthur had previously publicly stated that both the state and local officials had overstepped their authority by restricting churches – something that he was indeed correct on as the 1st Amendment of the Bill of Rights explicitly protects churches against government interference. Initially, LA County sought to shut down the church via the use of a restraining order, but this was struck down by the LA County Superior Court. To counter, the revoking of the parking lot was enacted.

According to Jenna Ellis, the attorney representing Grace Community Church, "The Democrats' message to Americans is clear – if you don't bow to every whim of tyranny, the government will come after you." MacArthur added, "We've all been suspicious of the fact that we've been meeting together now for weeks and weeks and weeks, and we don't know anyone who's ill. Nobody in our congregation has ever been to the hospital with this." He went on, "...it's not a surprise to me that, in the midst of all this deception, the great effort that is going on is to shut down churches that preach the gospel."[12]

Reverend Dennis Jackman of Community United Methodist Church in Pasadena, Maryland fought similar government harassment. His church was cited by the Anne Arundel County Department of Health for a health code violation after the pastor (who was alone in the church) opened the church door for a health department official's unannounced visit without wearing a mask. As a result, he was told that the church was not in full compliance with the local restrictions, and that the church would be deemed an "unsafe facility" and "closed until the state of emergency has been terminated." The citation also warned of imprisonment of up to one year and/or a fine of up to $5000.

And this was *despite* the fact that the church *had* been following all county guidelines for coronavirus. He'd been preaching his sermons *from the bed of a pickup truck* in the church parking lot.

According to Reverend Jackman, "I was in my office alone, without a mask on, and heard someone at the locked door of the church. I was not expecting anyone, so I went to see who was trying to get in the church. Immediately after answering the door, I went to my desk and put on my mask, but the health official seemed intent on finding something worthy of a citation."

The church had also been reported to officials for engaging in such "unsafe" practices as hand shaking, high fives, and fist bumps.

There were other churches targeted in Maryland as well. Calvary Baptist Church in Dundalk, Maryland faced similar unconstitutional threats from the Baltimore County Department of Health and Human Services in the form of a cease-and-desist letter saying that the church could be fined up to $5000 if the church continued to have in-person services in defiance of the Governor Larry Hogan's executive orders. For further perspective on this, keep in mind that within a week prior of the attack against Reverend Jackman, Governor Hogan had signed an executive order that released multitudes of prisoners throughout the state of Maryland due to COVID concerns.[13]

Does this not lead one to wonder as to whether or not the health officials are sincere in their "fear" that the churches of their state are hotspots of disease? What benefit does it serve to society to release *true* prisoners while criminalizing church members? Is there a deeper agenda involved?

Governor Cuomo and NYC Mayor de Blasio seem to have taken a particular interest in their city's Jewish population. The night after Joe Biden's "win" for the presidential election, thousands celebrated in the streets of New York City with no harassment from the local police or health department. A Jewish woman who owned a pottery shop in Brooklyn was caught on camera being harassed by a police officer over a COVID-related violation, however.[14]

That's not the only instance of such in NYC either. Video has also caught police officers responding to the funeral of a Jewish rabbi after they received reports that there were "too many" cars parked in front of a particular building.

An urgent appeal was also put out by the New York Health Department for staffers to go to Rockland and Orange counties – both of which have very large communities of ultra-orthodox Jewish communities who had defied "safety" protocols - to "perform COVID-19 community outreach and enforce mask and social distancing protocols...". Enforcement officers who did such were eligible for overtime pay.[15]

It was November 8, 2020, that a large Jewish wedding took place within New York City. And it was *large*. We're talking 7000 people. Imagine the caterer's bill. Despite the married couple not sending out invitations and having no such paper trail to their wedding, they were somehow found out and ratted out to the "authorities". In turn, Mayor de Blasio stated on November 23, 2020, that City Hall was fining the synagogue $15,000, and that there "could be additional consequences quite soon as well." The synagogue also received a cease and desist order and were told that should they engage in other "illegal" activities in the future that they risked being shut down permanently.

The New York Post jumped in on the nonsense, stating that people at the wedding were "stomping, dancing, and singing at the top of their lungs without a mask in sight." Can you imagine people *singing*? How dangerous! Governor Cuomo furthered the situation by stating the event was both "illegal" and "disrespectful", apparently forgetting that violating human rights – as protected within the First Amendment of the Bill of Rights – is in fact illegal, and therefore, disrespectful.[16]

Canada saw similar religious persecution throughout 2020. After meeting in-person on November 22, the Church of God at Steinbach in Manitoba received a $5000 fine for violating COVID regulations. In response, they held a drive-in church service on November 29. However, even *this* was deemed "unsafe" by the authorities. When churchgoers showed up for their service that morning, they were met by a significant police presence who wouldn't let them even drive into the church parking lot, even though the service was going to be held with congregation members in their cars with the windows up. In response, the congregation lined the highway in front of the church with their cars.

The provincial government had declared that drive-in services were not allowed either. According to Manitoba's chief provincial public health officer, Dr. Brent Roussin, this is because drive-in services are dangerous, and people just need to stay at home.

Pastor Henry Hildebrandt had a bit to say about that. "Make no mistake, this is not about a virus," he stated, going on to mention that churches "have been singled out" in the lockdowns while pot shops, liquor stores, and fast-food joints had been deemed "essential" by the government. He went on to say that the violation of the churchgoer's "right to religious freedom and peaceful assembly in the Canadian Constitution" is not something Christians follow in "blind obedience".

"On Sunday morning, people in this province interacted at Walmart, Costco, and other retailers. The same thing happened at the local liquor store, cannabis dispensaries, and the list goes on. Yet, it is our faith community that is singled out for public criticism, media attention, and visits by the RCMP, Manitoba Public Health, and local bylaw enforcement."[17]

Samuel Adams – one of the greatest Americans to ever have lived – summed this up perfectly within his paper "The Rights of the Colonists as Men". He said, "As neither reason requires nor religion permits the contrary, every man living in or out of a state of civil society has a right peaceably and quietly to worship God according to the dictates of his conscience."[18]

If such truly is the case – and it is undoubtedly so – then what right has any government worker have to ensure that citizens cannot do so? In stopping citizens from doing so, are they acting within the bounds of their authority, or have they turned themselves into nothing more than a bunch of thugs with badges?

What Can We Glean?

   Public health needs to be kept about public health. It can very easily be used as a dangerous weapon, in a sense being something of a policy machine capable of mass destruction. Freedoms die when public health policy is wielded as a sword by the unjust and petty. Americans need to understand this and to hold public health authorities responsible for the decisions that they make.

   Checks and balances need to be instituted once more, and the best way that I see such of taking place is to once more permit only the Legislative branch of the American government to craft laws as is stated within the US Constitution. To permit any other agency to create regulations with the exact same penalties as laws is to violate the US Constitution. It is to permit the growth of a nightmare.

13

Peoples' Response

With the mess that was the year 2020 it will be interesting for the reader to study what the people of the world's response was to the massive infarctions against basic human rights. Public policy creation is a subject that every public health student must be literate in, and the ability to create sound policy that is scientifically sound, feasible, cost-effective, and that does not violate human rights is fundamental to this knowledge.

When one does not listen to these basic logical needs for government policy, a number of things are bound to happen. They've happened in every single instance throughout history. One of the first things that we saw was massive unrest in the population at large. This was due to a large number of reasons. Black Lives Matter and Antifa protested and engaged in mob rule throughout the country, beating those who were white, of a different political persuasion, or who were deemed to be "bourgeoisie" to a pulp. Public health policy shut down peoples' abilities to earn a living, throwing millions throughout the US onto government assistance. Food banks commonly had lines of up to 12 hours as a result. People were arrested for otherwise mundane activities such as surfing or showing their face in public.

And what did we see happen?

Increase in Firearms, Ammo, and Body Armor Sales

As a result of all this – as well as political fears of a socialist/communist uprising with the potential incoming of a Joe Biden/Kamala Harris presidency – gun sales absolutely went through the roof within the United States. According to the National Shooting Sports Foundation, there was more than 2.5 million *new* gun owners in America in the first half of 2020 alone. Palmetto State Armory, a budget-friendly firearms manufacturer noticed a similar trend with a massive surge in first-time gun owners. In particular, PSA reported a surge of interest in anything AR-15 or defense related as well.

The National Instant Criminal Background Check System saw 3.9 million background checks in June of 2020 alone, the highest number reported ever since the system began back in 1998. And that doesn't even begin to cover the amount of firearms that were sold or built throughout the US without ever having been registered or had paperwork attached to them. How many were 3D printed?

Within the United States, ammunition sales skyrocketed as well, with an ammo shortage sweeping the nation and the market price of ammo going for as much as 3x what it had been going for just a year prior. According to Google, search results for the phrase "buy ammo" spiked over 900% from January 2020 to March 2020, and the phrase "best handgun" spiked over 300% during that same time frame.

Sales of body armor increased exponentially as well. Alex Lind, marketing manager of AR500 Armor, a company that specializes in body armor, reported that as of July 15 his company's sales had gone up 450% since the same time a year ago. Google Trends noticed similar results with the phrase "body armor" spiking over 130% from January to early June.[1]

Other companies that sell body armor throughout the US reported similar results. Brad Pedell, a body armor dealer in New York City noted that his sales of body armor had jumped over 80% compared to 2019. He gave the main reason as being unrest throughout his city, most of his buyers being from the Bronx and Brooklyn.

In addition, Pedell noted that many of his customers have become very standoffish regarding *why* they are actually buying the body armor to begin with. Refusal to give details as to why they are making such a purchase has become common, though it can be deduced this is because people value their privacy and don't trust the government with the knowledge of who has body armor and where.[2]

Decrease in College Enrollment

Colleges saw a massive decrease in the number of students across the nation as well. George Washington University saw its enrollment drop by 17% in 2020 compared to 2019. This university wasn't alone, however. The National Association of College and University Business Officers found that fully 67% of colleges across the nation expect enrollment to decrease significantly.[3]

This is most likely due to fears of COVID-19, and the fear of being in places with large numbers of people. One potential benefit to this, however, could be the lack of access to the public at large that communists will have for spreading their agenda. It has long been noted that a sizeable portion – if not the majority – of academia throughout the United States has been firm evangelists of collectivism and agnosticism towards America's youth. Without access to new recruits, their strength diminishes.

For further research into this, I highly recommend reading *None Dare Call it Treason, The Naked Communist,* or *The Naked Socialist.*

As of this writing, a number of colleges and universities throughout the US are now mandating that all of their students possess a vaccination passport for COVID before attending classes there. I believe it is reasonable to expect attendance to continue to drop off for colleges in the future as students refuse to apply for such paperwork.

Outright Defiance

There were a number of cases of mayors, sheriffs, police departments, and governors explicitly stating that they would not follow or enforce "laws" deemed unconstitutional that were sent from a higher authority.

South Dakota's Governor Kristi Noem was one of the more outspoken examples of such, with her statements that if Joe Biden took over the presidency, that he would not have the authority to impose the nationwide mask mandate on state governments that he had long since espoused. According to Noem, she trusted her residents "to make wise and well-informed decisions for themselves and their families" instead of having the government tell citizens what they must do under penalty of punishment.[4]

Fulton County Sheriff Richard Giardino had a similar response to New York's Governor Cuomo when new restrictions were announced in time for Thanksgiving 2020. The new restrictions said that gatherings of people could not exceed 10 people, *including* at private residencies. This made it illegal under penalty of law throughout the state of

New York for families to visit loved ones during Thanksgiving. Giardino responded to this blatant overreach of state government by explicitly stating that his deputies would not enforce Cuomo's unconstitutional decree.[5]

Cuomo responded by saying, "I don't believe as a law enforcement officer you have a right to pick and choose what laws you will enforce," going on to state than an executive order "is a law". "There's a law, and you have to enforce the law, or don't call yourself a law enforcement officer."[6]

Perhaps one shouldn't call themselves an American if they behave like a Russian communist either.

Mass Exodus

Due to both anger from government overreach, and fear of overcrowding, large cities throughout the world saw a mass exodus as the populace sought refuge in more rural geographies. Sales of RVs, backpacking equipment, and the like saw a huge spike throughout 2020 as people sought to escape from the presence of others. This saw its biggest push in the beginning of 2020 when fear of COVID was at its peak, and uncertainty as to just how bad the disease was going to be ran rampant. As those fears were quelled as more statistics became available, this author would argue that the majority of the exoduses were due to a desire to be free.

Paris saw this October 30, 2020. French president Macron mandated a second national lockdown to begin on this day, and as a result, *hundreds* of miles of traffic jams occurred on all routes out of the famous city. Macron's order required all residents to stay at home at all times other than for what *he* had deemed "essential work" or for medical reasons. The French media noted that the jams were truly record breaking and noticed similar mass exoduses in the French cities of Lyon and Bordeaux. According to Le Parisien, "there was more than 430 miles of gridlock traffic in the city by 6pm."[7]

California likewise saw a mass exodus of its population due to the miserable living conditions that had been created there (in many cases as a result of their own voting patterns). So many Californians began to leave that politicians there began to grow frantic about the potential loss of tax revenue. As potential legislation began to float around about requiring all Californian emigrants to pay 10 years in state taxes first even more Californians packed their bags.

The end result was an influx of Californians throughout the rest of America. Texas, Montana, and many other predominantly conservative states suddenly had an influx of liberals.

14

Hold on a Minute

"It is so true, that the Socialists look upon mankind as a subject for social experiments, that if, by chance, they are not quite certain of the success of these experiments, they will request a portion of mankind, as a subject to experiment upon." – Frederic Bastiat[1]

Any outlandish or strange decision that government decides to make in the interest of public health should initially be screened through the people first. Otherwise, one can very quickly end up with situations where public health authorities rubber stamp what can only be described as Jurassic Park-esque scenarios where the potential ramifications could be huge.

One of the chief examples of such we saw throughout 2020 was with Floridian authorities coming to the conclusion that they needed to release millions of genetically modified mosquitoes into the wild as part of an *experiment*.

On August 18, the Monroe County Mosquito Control District gave the go-ahead for the release of 750 million genetically modified mosquitoes into the Florida Keys starting in the year 2021. The mosquitoes were created by the British company Oxitec and were approved for use by the Environmental Protection Agency within the US in May of 2020. Even the Centers for Disease Control and the Florida Department of Health rubber stamped Oxitec's GM mosquitoes.[2]

The purpose of this experiment was to see if these genetically altered mosquitoes (where the males were called OX5034) could prove to be a safer alternative to spraying insecticides throughout the state in order to control local populations of the mosquito *Aedes aegypti. Aedes* are known for spreading yellow fever, Zika virus, and chikungunya.

Typically, male mosquitoes only eat nectar, while it's the females who feast on human and animal blood. OX5034 was created to ensure the death of all larval female mosquitoes which bite and transmit disease. In theory, this would then lead to the extinction of Aedes aegypti.

Oxitec claims that the OX5034 is perfectly safe, with Nathan Rose, the director of regulatory affairs there stating, "We have shown that the release of mosquitoes in a neighborhood results in 95% suppression compared to areas with no release."[3]

The problems from such a decision are many. To begin with, our environment at large is a system. What happens when one removes just one part of it? Beekeepers have long stated that the removal of honeybees from society could have a devastating effect on the entire field of agriculture – leading in the end to harvests that are a fraction of what they were prior. What happens when you remove mosquitoes completely from the environment? What purposes do they fulfill that we either currently aren't aware of, or currently underestimate? How many species such as bats, birds, and frogs, do they currently feed – who also serve vital roles within the environment as a whole – and who would sequentially grow to be extinct due to our hubris in deciding that we simply must exterminate all mosquitoes.

History does not look kindly on the examples it can show of mankind doing such. The introduction of snakeheads, Japanese beetles, kudzu, and numerous other forms of wildlife has wreaked havoc on native populations of flora and fauna. What happens when one willfully removes one species entirely?

What about the neighboring states and counties that don't wish to have genetically modified mosquitoes flying about their neighborhoods? Mosquitoes haven't been noted to respect political boundaries, and the release of 750 million mosquitoes will most certainly result in their spread to neighboring counties surrounding Monroe County, Florida. Do neighboring regions not have a say on the public health policies that will affect them – and in an unknown manner – by default? Most certainly mosquitoes are vectors of disease. Most certainly it can be argued that the regular spraying of insecticides could have negative health effects for both humans and the environment. But is releasing hordes of GMOs the answer?

How much research has been done on this as a solution? Are there potential mutations that are possible that could wreak unintended consequences on both the environment as a whole and on mankind? What happens if we discover that GMO mosquitoes are prime petri dishes for strange mutations of viruses? Who wants to be bitten by a engineered mosquito? There are simply too many unknowns for any public health official to have enough hubris to decide that releasing GMO mosquitoes on his populace is a wise idea.

The point is that governments should not make decisions that affect others outside of their jurisdiction lightly. While it can always be argued "Well, we're helping reduce their mosquito population as well!", the point remains that surrounding communities are now going to see an influx of potential Frankenstein monsters that they are completely powerless to stop.

In many ways, it's akin to a city dumping all of their sewage into a river. All of the downstream communities will be impacted by such a decision, yet there will be little to nothing that they can do about it. When it's a massive experiment though – the first of its kind – and the potential ramifications could be terrifying, there needs to be an extreme degree of hesitation involved.

Further examples of such can be seen by Bill Gates' plan to blot out the sun in order to allegedly reduce global warming. While it sounds like something out of a science fiction movie, Bill Gates did indeed have plans to inject some form of haze-creating dust up into the stratosphere that would supposedly greatly reduce the amount of UV radiation that hit the earth.

Once more we see this basic principle at work: the notion that mankind is worthy of experimentation despite his protests to the contrary "for his own good".

What could be the potential consequences of darkening the sun? Is this an action that solely affects a small community that has voted for it, or is this an action that could potentially affect billions?

If we look back on a smaller level we see the same type of mindset taking place in Colorado. The Rocky Mountains effectively separate Colorado into two halves: the east and the west. The east half of Colorado is predominantly big cities and has an incredibly strong collectivist presence. In contrast, the western half of Colorado is more rural, and is a more freedom-friendly part of the state.

It was in 2020 that environmental activists on the east half of Colorado voted for the release of wolves on the west half of Colorado. The argument for such was that the wolves were needed because their populations were dropping too low. The people on the west side of Colorado protested against such a decision vehemently. Being largely an agrarian society, they argued that the release of wolves would cost them potentially millions of dollars in lost lambs, calves, and other livestock, not to mention the potential risk to their children who enjoyed playing outside.

But for the eastern half of Colorado these were the useless ramblings of out-of-touch and selfish individuals who needed to be taught a lesson. The bill passed and wolves were released on the western side of Colorado.

Yet again, we see people voting for something that has incredible potential to be destructive but for those that are far away. If one truly wants wolves to be released upon society, why not release them on your own turf? It's rather convenient to not have to worry about wolves in your own neighborhood, is it not? What can be said for the man that is willing to subject other men to a danger that he is not willing to face himself?

Government authorities should remember that the sole reason that they are in office – the sole reason that government exists in the first place – is to protect the rights of individuals. To expose others to very present risks is not only unwise but unjust.

15

That's Not Your Decision to Make

"The modern politicians....divide mankind into two parts. Men in general....form the first; the politician himself forms the second, which is by far the most important. In fact, they begin by supposing that men are devoid of any principle of action, and of any means of discernment in themselves; that they have no initiative; that they are inert matter, passive particles, atoms without impulse; at best a vegetation indifferent to its own mode of existence, susceptible of assuming, from an exterior will and hand an infinite number of forms, more or less symmetrical, artistic, and perfected. Moreover, every one of these politicians does not hesitate to assume that he himself is, under the names of organizer, discoverer, legislator, institutor or founder, this will and hand, this universal initiative, this creative power, whose sublime mission it is to gather together these scattered materials, that is, men, into society." – Frederic Bastiat[1]

Government is created to serve the people, and anytime that it attempts to make a decision that it has no right to make, its citizens are victim of an unlawful encroachment on their inherent rights. The reason that constitutions are written is to create limitations on *government*, not on people. As Ayn Rand pointed out, "A government official may do nothing except that which is legally *permitted*."[2]

To be a government official – to be a public health officer – is *not* to have a blank check from which one can make unlimited withdrawals against the natural human rights of a populace. It is those who argue against this who are some of the most dangerous advocates of tyranny and all that it entails (e.g. genocide).

Ayn Rand further went on to say, "The source of the government's authority is 'the consent of the governed.' This means that the government is not the *ruler*, but the servant or *agent* of the citizens; it means that the government as such has no rights except the rights *delegated* to it by the citizens for a specific purpose."[2] Thus, any action that a government agent attempts to take (or does in actuality take) which is beyond his scope of authority is not only a breach of authority, but criminal, and should be treated as such. For example, in 2020 a police officer forced a man to lick a public urinal.[3] While the police officer was the government agent, and while the police officer did have the capability to use lethal force, did that police officer have the right to force a man to lick a public urinal? Does that fall within the bounds of his realm of authority? If one says that it does not (as any reasonable human being should), then that would mean that the man would have been correct to resist against the use of force to get him to do so.

Government has no power other than that which is delegated to it. Any overstepping of this boundary is criminal. This is not what's taught throughout public health graduate schools however, and I believe that this is a great part of the problem. It's those who are being trained to be the next generation of public health officers who are being taught that they can, in essence, do whatever they want. Take for example, this quote from a prominent public health graduate textbook on public health administration:

"The police powers represent the state's authority to further the goal of all government, which is to promote the general welfare of society. Police powers can be defined as: the inherent authority of the state (and, throughout delegation, local government) to enact laws and promulgate regulations to protect, preserve, and promote the health, safety, morals, and general welfare of the people. To achieve these communal benefits, the state retains the power to restrict, within federal and state constitutional limits, private interests – personal interests in liberty, autonomy, privacy, and association, as well as economic interests in freedom of contract and uses of property."

The text goes on: "Thus, government has inherent power to interfere with personal interests in autonomy, liberty, privacy, and association, as well as economic interest in ownership and uses of private property."

And on:

"Police powers exercised by the states include vaccination, isolation and quarantine, inspection of commercial and residential premises, abatement of unsanitary conditions or other nuisances, and regulation of air and surface water contaminants, as well as restriction on the public's access to polluted areas, standards for pure food and drinking water, extermination of vermin, fluoridization of municipal water supplies, and licensure of physicians and other healthcare professionals."[4]

There are a number of rather scary logical conclusions that can be reached by such a stance. Imagine a world where police powers back up vaccination. If you believe that a particular vaccine is dangerous, refusing to take it, you are now a criminal and will be treated as such. This is to say that government has the right to pin you to the ground as your surrounded by men with guns leveled at your head, and a needle is jabbed into your arm.

Nowhere within the US Constitution do I see that power given to any government authority. You can undoubtedly find other problems with such quotes. And it is because of this type of logic – because of this belief that public health officials *of necessity* must be dictatorial that throughout 2020 we saw mayors, sheriffs, governors, and others attempt to step into decisions that they had no legal standing to make.

One such example comes from lawmakers deciding that they had the authority to decide which medical procedures a patient could undergo, and which they could not. During November of 2020, Ohio lawmakers threatened to postpone elective surgeries due to COVID-19. Republican Governor Mike DeWine of Ohio stated that due to new cases "overwhelming the system" that "we'll need to make more decisions about how we triage."[5]

He said this despite both his and his lawmaker's having absolutely *zero* authority to engage in medical triage. Since when do governors have any say in who can undergo an elective procedure and who cannot? Does your governor have the right to determine whether or not your father can undergo his hemorrhoid surgery, whether you can get your hernia repaired, or whether your son can get his knee surgery? Who wants to place that much power in a single individual?

Part of the very nature of a free society is that the individual has the right to purchase what he desires and when he desires to do so. Obviously, this does not apply to prostitution or drugs which literally turn one into a monster (e.g. bath salt designer drugs), but for all else, the basic principle of laissez faire applies. The more the government gets involved – particularly in instances of personal health and medical decisions – the less free a society is. And there can be some rather terrifying ramifications when government decides it has the authority to make such decisions and is left unchecked by the people whom it was created to serve.

What about when the government decides what you can eat and what you cannot? Though this most certainly happened in 2020, it actually happened long before that as well. Philadelphia's soda tax and New York City's similar laws made it illegal to actually buy certain sizes of soda.[6] You could buy as much alcohol, tobacco, or other items as you like, but the option to buy a particular size of Pepsi at a gas station was made illegal. All in the name of public health.

However, 2020 gave us examples of this as well. Both California and New York forced restaurants and bars to only serve alcohol with meals in the name of helping to "stop the spread". For many of these businesses – particularly bars – serving alcohol by itself is the main source of revenue. Though I am not entirely sure about the thought process behind such a decision, I believe that the reason the forcing of alcohol to be sold with meals was made was to decrease the number of customers that utilized a restaurant or bar. Can there be any other explanation?

Aside from the clear government overreach here, with the state decision that you don't *need* that many customers, is it not scary when the government decides that it has the authority to decide if you can go out and buy a beer and if you cannot?

In order to work around this ridiculous restriction, many of these affected businesses added special menu items so that their patrons could still buy an alcoholic beverage without having to also spend money on a lavish meal. Items such as pretzel bites, hot wings, and similar small items were added for a marginal cost so that customers could still do business with their desired bar/restaurant without that business having to fear of running afoul of the "law".

California's governor Newsom then decreed that buffalo chicken wings were not a meal.

He further decreed that "any small portion of a dish that may constitute a main course when it is not served in a full portion or when it is intended for sharing in small portions" were banned as well. In New York, Cuomo decreed that "the lowest level of substantive food were sandwiches".[7]

Once more, a man powerful enough to determine that sandwiches are the lowest level of substantive food is a man powerful enough to determine virtually any other aspect of your life that he wakes up and decides to as well. Such power is not vested in governors, mayors, or anybody else in a political office throughout the United States of America, and not only should not be complied with, but should be resisted by the people as well.

Even within the realm of online learning we saw blatant levels of government overreach where they attempted to tell people what they could and could not do *within their own home*. Shelby County, Tennessee made it against the rules for kids to eat or drink while attending online classes. Keep in mind that these kids are taking these classes often times from their kitchen tables. Thus, the state has decreed that during a particular time of the day you can no longer eat or drink *in your own home*.[8]

Understandably, a businessman is unlikely to want to be eating a cheeseburger while he is on a telecom interview with a potential partner in India. However, many times such a business call would take place while both men are at their work offices. Rarely, if ever, would such a conference call be conducted while both men were in their own homes. That being said, would either party likely object to the others drinking out of a glass of water? How does it negatively affect children's learning ability if they eat a snack while they are attending an online math lecture? Does a public health official, or any official for that matter, have that kind of power?

What about the power to deny you access to water, air conditioning, heat, and electricity? Does a politician have the power to grant or deny access to any of those to you? One would think not, right? However, those in California apparently thought otherwise. In what was a rather chilling statement on August 5, 2020, LA mayor Eric Garcetti announced that he was authorizing the city to shut off the utilities to homes where "large" parties or gatherings were held.[9]

Imagine what this implies. Not only does it indicate that there will be police officers strolling the streets to count the number of cars in private driveways and looking through windows to see if they can see more than what *they've* deemed "appropriate", but it also means a politician has decided he has the authority to determine how many people that you can or cannot have in your home. And this isn't talking about violating fire code regulations either. We're not talking about attempting to squeeze 300 people into a mobile home. We're talking about a gathering of 15 people. You do *that* and you risk not being able to have heat in your home in the dead of winter. One need only a couple seasons' worth of news cycles to understand that people still die from exposure to the elements when there are extremes of heat or cold. Even in the US. So when Garcetti threatened such, he truly threatened the lives of the constituents whom he decided to treat as little children.

Samuel Adams had something to say about this. He said, "The legislative cannot justly assume to itself a power to rule by extempore arbitrary decrees; but it is bound to see that justice is dispensed, and that the rights of the subjects be decided by promulgated standing, and known laws, and authorized independent judges; that is, independent, as far as possible, of prince and people. There should be one rule of justice for rich and poor, for the favorite at court, and the countryman at the plough."[10]

Other Founding Fathers pointed out similar. In his essay "Common Sense", Thomas Paine said, "...in America the LAW is king."[11] It is not men in the US who are able to rule with an iron fist, but instead the *law* that dictates what a man can and cannot do. This same principle applies to those who are in positions of government office as well. And the supreme law of the land within the United States is the Constitution. There can be no law within the US that is in violation of the US Constitution. As prior court cases (Marbury v. Madison) have decided, any law which is in contradiction to the US Constitution is automatically null and void. It cannot exist for the sole reason that the Constitution says that it cannot!

As such, you cannot make a law that prohibits freedom of speech. Why? Because such is protected by the First Amendment within the US Constitution. Any law that is set up that is in contradiction with the First Amendment is automatically null and void according to US law, and thus is not a law in the first place.

Furthermore, we have to consider how the American system of government works. Within the US we have three branches of government: the legislative, executive, and judicial branches. Each branch has very specific roles and abilities. One of these roles is the creation of new laws. The authority for such is bestowed upon the legislative branch, and no other branch has the right to invade the domain of the legislative branch in order to craft new laws.

According to the US Constitution, there is a very formal process for the crafting of new laws, with Congress being required to act in order to do such. Now you have to ask yourself, did your local public health department go through Congress to pass its laws? Can it be argued that regulations are not laws? If you're going to potentially fine, imprison, or do other punitive measures against me with police assistance should I not comply with what you say, can it be argued that you've set into place anything other than a law? Do police get involved in matters that do not involve the law? Regardless of the name involved for your decisions, if you are able to involve the police or heavy fines to punish somebody for breaking it, you *have* created a law, whether you will call it by its rightful name or not.

So the question is, does a public health official have the right to create these laws in the first place according to the US Constitution? Did the legislative branch give them the authority to do so? If so, did the legislative branch have the right to delegate that power to a further branching in the first place?

16

Lack of Healthcare Access

Quite possibly one of the most egregious failures in public health policy is in the forced removal of access to healthcare. This author witnessed this firsthand throughout hospitals in his state. As this author was entering a local doctor's office, patients with a history of cardiac disease were denied access to a doctor if they were older than 70 years old. I witnessed firsthand as a secretary told an older woman that no, she could not go to see the doctor because she was older than 70, and thus, it was unsafe for her to do so.

The woman was visibly upset, saying that she "felt as if she was being thrown to the wolves." If the woman is willing to take the "risk" and visit the doctor, and the doctor is willing to see her, why does hospital administration feel that they need to step in and deny this? Is it riskier for a patient with a history of disease to not be able to see their doctor, or is it riskier for them to see the doctor – who is in full PPE garb – for fears of contracting a virus with a 99.97% survival rate?

Is it morally justifiable to deny people access to healthcare due to fears that the person (who desires to enter the facility, regardless of the "risks") could end up getting sick?

I would argue the answer is a definitive no. If we are to see a drastic rise in deaths from various diseases and chronic conditions over the next 1-2 years, I would argue that it is largely due to idiotic decisions such as this one.

It is most certainly one thing for a doctor to refuse to perform an experimental procedure on a patient who desires the experimental procedure if the doctor does not feel that it would be in the patient's best interest to do so. This could be due to the doctor not being familiar with the procedure or thinking that the procedure's risks well outweigh the potential for rewards. It's for this reason that many doctors are hesitant to perform experimental surgeries on very young patients who are not faced with some type of terminal illness/situation. I myself have done this with patients. If I do not feel that performing a certain therapy exercise would be beneficial – and in fact, that it would be harmful – I will not prescribe it.

Imagine the man who just had a shoulder replacement wanting his therapist to prescribe bench pressing. The therapist could tell the man there's no way that was going to happen just yet – that to do so would be unsafe – yet despite the patient's pleas, the therapist holds his ground. There is a 100% risk the therapist knows about that *will* result in injury, and in such a case, to prescribe that treatment would be morally wrong.

However, it becomes quite a different situation if the patient is terminal, desires the experimental treatment, and literally has nothing to lose from the situation.

What if that's not what we're talking about? What if we're living in a constant state of fear over what *could* happen? What if we're denying access to healthcare for a patient not because of the definitive consequences, but because there is some astronomically small chance that something bad could happen? Is that fair to do to the patient even if they are willing to brave the risks?

Is it right to turn away a patient for fear that they could end up catching the flu? If this were the case, wouldn't doctor's offices across the nation have to completely close down every flu season in order to keep people with sprained wrists and troubles with their blood glucose from potentially catching the flu from a sick patient? Can you see why this is so ridiculous?

What if the argument is pushed even further? Do you as a doctor have the right to refuse medical care to a patient because they are not vaccinated or won't wear a mask? Why is it that for years doctors would take their own safety upon *themselves* in treating homeless gay men that likely had AIDS, yet now, all of a sudden, we have doctors that refuse to treat patients because they don't have an (unscientific) mask strapped across their face? Why has the burden of safety suddenly shifted to the patient?

To do so is to ask the gunshot wound patient to quit bleeding out of their abdomen, as they might unwillingly be spreading some form of infectious agent across the room. Yet there are those in current society who are more than happy to apply the same sort of logic to simply walking through an emergency room door.

"We're sorry, sir, but you can't come in here without a mask."

That's a rather twisted world to live in, when you can't walk into an emergency room *with an emergency,* mind you, because you don't have a piece of cloth across your face, is it not? Videos actually surfaced out of the United Kingdom in 2021 illustrating such logic at work though. In one video, a man with a broken neck was denied treatment because he refused to be tested for COVID prior to the procedure. At this time, the UK had "quarantine facilities" complete with guards, barbed wire, and tall fences for those who had been deemed 'positive'. They were nothing short of prisons. Likewise, there was a lot of talk at this time of people getting *brain* infections from COVID-testing swabs (several children actually ended up with such), and discussion coming out regarding nanotechnology being preinserted on COVID-testing swabs.

While some of this may sound far-fetched to readers, the point remains: you have the right to deny medical treatments should you desire to do so. It is your body, not the doctor's, and you have the right to decide what happens with your original piece of property. What difference does it make to be tested anyway either? All through my training, I was taught that you take maximum precautions with each patient. To act as if each person coming through that door had AIDS. Would a positive COVID test cause the doctor to behave any differently towards the patient? Why not just wear the mask and gear you would likely wear anyways and get the job done?

This comes down to *philosophy* once more. Man should be responsible for his own safety, and this does not come at the expense of intruding on the rights of others, particularly in a manner of saying that another man must have some type of substance injected into *his* body, that a man must wear a mask across *his* face, so that you can feel safe. To argue for such is to claim that you have mastership over all of the people around you.

As John Stuart Mills pointed out, "The only freedom which deserves the name, is that of pursuing our own good in our own way, so long as we do not attempt to deprive others of theirs, or impede their efforts to obtain it. Each is the proper guardian of his own health, whether bodily, or mental and spiritual. Mankind are greater gainers by suffering each other to live as seems good to themselves, than by compelling each to live as seems good to the rest."[1]

Chapter 16 – Lack of Healthcare Access

In America we live in the land of the free (at least it once was), and thus, you have no right to infringe upon the rights of others. To do so is to be a rouge, regardless of what your position is. If you can refuse service to somebody because they don't have a mask, a vaccine passport, or the like, would you be ok if they did the same to you in their field of work? It is likely that the doctor who refused healthcare access to a young man with a broken arm and no vaccination paperwork would be upset when the father – a plumber – showed up for an emergency backed up sewer line, discovered who the doctor was, and then refused to provide service.

What would happen if a white American were to refuse permitting people of brown color into his grocery store? The public would be irate! The man would likely face death threats and witness the burning down of his store.

And yet, we are rapidly moving towards being a nation where we tolerate, expect, and enforce such actions against those who are not of the same mind as us.

I would argue that the only lack of healthcare access that is justified is based upon cost alone. Plastic surgery is easily considered to fall under the umbrella term of healthcare. If a woman wants a breast enlargement surgery, yet cannot afford such, to deny her access to that form of healthcare is justified. However, to deny her access to such when she can afford it, when such a surgery would not negatively affect her health, and when the doctor is more than willing to perform the surgery on other patients, would not be. If the surgeon denied the woman access to the surgery simply because of her skin color or nationality – neither of which were factors that would negatively affect the surgery – then there would very quickly prove to be a legal and moral issue.

So how can we then argue that to deny people access to healthcare because of vaccination status, masking status, age, or abysmally small risk of infection are right and proper?

17

Management of Public Fear

One of the chief concerns that seems to cause politicians to make stupid decisions is the fear of public panic. We heard this throughout the beginning of 2020, of how the most dangerous thing that we had to fear was fear itself, and that it was fear which was more dangerous than the virus. The underlying message here - that the *public* cannot be trusted with the facts – while those in office *can* – is condescending to the extreme. Government should be as transparent as possible. There is most certainly a need for secrecy when it comes to wartime information or other data that could be dangerous to the nation to be public knowledge (e.g. nuclear secrets). But to block information regarding a virus or other infectious disease is to be part of the problem, not part of the solution.

That being said, the mainstream media pulled a complete 180 as 2020 went along, and it came to almost seem as if the MSM made it their job not to inform, but to *spread* as much fear as possible. Fear makes people do stupid things. It makes people become different people.

It was fear that made a Long Island, NY man threaten to shoot people at a *children's* yeshiva camp because he didn't think that the kids were properly socially distancing. Nicola Pelle, the complainer, had actually called police because the children at the Yeshiva Ketano of Long Island were "playing and not social distancing" nor wearing masks. Cops were apparently sent out to check out the scene, but Pelle felt the need to call again because he didn't feel as if the cops were arriving to the scene fast enough. This time he said, "If I gotta go out there with a freaking machine gun and shoot all these people, I will." He was arrested.[1]

This is the degree of fear that the media stoked throughout 2020. When threatening to machine gun down children because they are playing on a playground becomes a viable alternative, something has gone wrong.

This author witnessed something similar to this via the NextDoor app. NextDoor is in essence a version of Facebook for a neighborhood to communicate with one another about suspicious persons, community events, and the like. One of the women within the author's neighborhood complained about the amount of shooting that was taking place near her rural home during the beginning of deer season. She complained that it was scaring her small dog, that she had moved to the South from New Jersey, that she had guns which she target practiced with as well, but that there was simply too much shooting happening in the woods around her. Her initial post garnered dozens of replies from neighbors who thought she was being unreasonable, and who told her to go back to New Jersey.

Her response was that those people with guns should use them to keep people from entering the local Food Lion without a mask. This is modern day society. Hunting and target practice are wrong (because they scare a *dog*) but using guns to threaten bodily harm against people who won't wear an ineffective face diaper to buy their groceries is completely warranted.

It wasn't just the media that was the culprit, however. The government itself was in every way complicit. What can be the point of turning the Empire State Building in NYC into a gigantic flashing red emergency beacon during the beginning of the pandemic?[2] What does that accomplish? How is that beneficial? This was nothing more than a move to stoke the fires of fear in the public's hearts.

Such actions nurture and cultivate fear, helping it to flourish. And when fear flourishes, people become monsters. Take the actions of Disney, for example. In August of 2020, a Pennsylvania family with a 7-year-old daughter with special needs traveled to Florida to visit the Magic Kingdom. They had pre-paid for their 8-day stay and had planned the trip for two years. For many, taking their children to the Magic Kingdom is considered a rite of passage – a essential part of childhood that cannot be bypassed without seriously doing a disfavor to the child.

However, after getting to the gates of the Magic Kingdom, workers told the father that his daughter could not enter the park without wearing a mask. This despite his daughter's inability to wear a mask. Workers responded that there were no exemptions. What class of human denies a little girl's ability to go to Disney World because she won't hide her face in public?

This wasn't the only Disney incident though. A 6-year-old autistic girl was asked to leave the Disney store in Ontario, Canada because she was unable to wear her mask properly. When questioned regarding their decision, a Disney representative said, "We regret the family was disappointed."[3]

As you can see, fear turns people into monsters. It robs people of their sense – of their humanity. That is why it is absolutely vital that public health authorities do everything in their power to take the following three steps.

First, they should be as transparent as possible. To not be so, is to assume that you are a special class of human above the rest of society. Treat people as adults, give them the facts, and then let them handle the information. Any attempts at shielding the truth *will* eventually be revealed to the public and when this happens, both you and your office will have lost all credibility. Any attempt from that point on to institute any policies or disseminate any information will be met with well-deserved scorn.

Secondly, do not willfully spread fear. There is most certainly a difference between fearmongering and telling the truth. If things are grim, then say so. But don't turn the most iconic building in your city into a giant flashing red beacon. That does nothing other than *spread* fear. Do not be afraid to tell the truth but use enough wisdom and discretion to do so in a manner that doesn't cultivate panic. While one can never completely eradicate panic, one can most certainly help to not spread it.

If America at large was notified that the Russians had just invaded Alaska – and that Alaska had fallen – there is going to be panic regardless of what you say. At some point, you have to leave people's actions up to them. You are not a babysitter.

Thirdly, don't act manipulative and *understand* when you're being manipulated. If there is data that it is readily apparent has been tinkered with, then don't disseminate it. To do so is to be a part of the problem, and is to further perpetuate a lie upon the American people (which, as we'll remember is a violation of the transparency the public deserves – you were not put in office as a *public servant* to lie).

Provided that the public health officer can keep these three points in mind, information will be disseminated to the public without a furthering of fearmongering.

18

Immigration/Travel/Boundaries

Let's perform another mind experiment, shall we? Let's say that there is an incredibly contagious and deadly respiratory agent that is spreading across the world. We don't really know anything about it. Where it came from (e.g. a lab/terrorist attack/etc.), what to treat it with, or any functioning epidemiology is all currently a mystery to us. All we really know is that it's deadly and that it seems to spread person-to-person. Whether that be through direct contact, droplets, or airborne particulates, we're not really sure. We just know that other people are dangerous at the moment.

Given such were the case, what do you have the right to do as the mayor/sheriff/town council of where you live? Your job is to protect and serve the citizens who elected you into office, is it not? If such is truly the case, do you have the duty to prevent the illness from reaching your community? For the sake of argument, let's say that you live on Bald Head Island off the coast of the Outer Banks in North Carolina. Bald Head Island is a very small community where a good portion of the homes are actually nothing more than vacation homes. The owners rent them out but live up much further north somewhere.

So here you are as the mayor of Bald Head Island, and where you live is naturally separated from the rest of the world. If you can simply keep people who may be sick from

214

visiting your island, there's no reason to believe that any of your citizens will ever come into contact with exactly whatever it is that's out there and causing such devastation. You have enough supplies to make it for quite some time (at least two months) without leaving the island. There's plenty of infrastructure on the island store-wise to provide basic goods. The island is largely uninhabited. And there's always the potential to fish for food.

If all of the above is the case, do you have the right – or even the duty – to shut off all transportation to and from your island? Doing so is easily done – all you have to do is to close down the ferry service and put your police force out to sea to keep any other boats from entering the island.

Such is the question that many communities faced throughout the beginning of 2020 as COVID-19 was spreading across the planet and there were more unknowns than there was knowledge. Trees were felled to block roads on islands in Maine in order to keep outsiders from getting in. In other locations, trees were felled to keep people from exiting their driveways after they were diagnosed with COVID.[1] Sheriffs set up roadblocks to an island off of the Outer Banks of North Carolina (*not* Bald Head Island, by the way) in order to keep their communities protected from the virus.[2]

But now the question remains: is such an action right or wrong? Is such an action a duty?

I believe that we can get a better grasp of what one is to do when one looks at the after effects of what happened with COVID-19. That one particular island in North Carolina faced a mountain of legal problems post-hoc. This author personally knows the owner of one of the vacation homes on that island. She detailed to me how she owned property there which she rented out a week at a time throughout the course of the year. Her beachfront property helped to provide her with a steady source of income throughout the year and was where she intended to live full-time after she retired in the near future. Living hours away from North Carolina, she let a local real estate office manage the vacation home for her.

Imagine her surprise when she was told by the real estate company that the sheriff department was not letting that week's renters onto the island. A family had driven the better half of a day from the Northeast to vacation at my friend's vacation home. Only to discover that they were not permitted on the island, and that if they tried, they would likely be arrested and thrown into jail. Furious, the family turned back around.

Things only grew more complicated.

Rightfully so, the vacationing family demanded their money back. They had paid in advance (as most vacation homes require) and had been prevented from using the home that they had paid for. According to the contract that they had signed, the only legal loophole that would prevent them from getting a refund would be if the island was evacuated due to a hurricane. Since such was not the case, they wanted their money back.

But the real estate company refused to give it to them.

They claimed (also rightfully so?) that since it had not been their fault that the island had been shut down by the sheriff that the money need to be sought not from their own hands, but instead at the hands of the local government. The renters then contacted my friend, seeking the money (several thousand dollars) from her directly instead. She also refused.

So what is to be done in such a situation? In this case, government intervention has created quite a mess. Had government never intervened here, there would have never been a problem. However, if we're to go back to our original mind experiment – that of a pandemic, airborne disease that we know nothing about – what can we say is the appropriate action? Are there actions that we can take that protect communities without violating human rights?

Let's examine such and see if we can come to any conclusions.

For starters, we do know that people are indeed dying from this disease. There's no question about such. This is truly a mass death scenario, and from initial reports, it looks like the lethality of this virus (?) is approximately 68%. If this virus reaches your community, it therefore very well may mean 68% of your population could end up dead (if everybody gets sick, of course. So, yes, that is a high number). You are the mayor of a community of 17,500 people, so this means you're potentially looking at a high estimate of 11,900 people dying.

As Ayn Rand has pointed out, you know that property rights are the most fundamental of all human rights. Once property rights are dismantled, all other rights of necessity will follow. Governments are created to protect peoples' individual rights. If you enact anything that goes against such, then you are violating the true purpose of government. However, you also know that part of this protection of peoples' individual rights is to protect from outside attack. This was why thousands of years' worth of history again and again show communities developing their own armies – to protect against outside attack.

Is it too far of a stretch to say that a deadly infectious disease is something of an outside aggressor? Again, there's no dispute here on the statistics. Everybody agrees that the threat is real, and nobody is questioning the data that is coming out of this. However, you also know that a great number of the properties within your community are owned by those who live nowhere near you. You're a tourist hotspot, and as a result a large number of northerners from current urban virus hotspots are likely to want to come to your location to "bug-out". If you let those northerners into your community they could very well bring disease with them.

What is the appropriate response?

Is it proper to completely shut down all borders, keeping even property owners from entering the inside after a set date? Or, do you only let property owners in, kicking all others out? Do you let in the friends and family of current property owners in your community? What if current residents have elderly parents on the outside that require daily care? Are they still allowed to tend to their parents, or are the parents brought back into the community as well?

While there most certainly are going to be disagreements with what I have to say on a very sticky issue – and admittedly, even inconsistencies on my part that I haven't discovered myself - here is my response. At the very least perhaps it will get you thinking through the appropriate means to handle such a situation.

I personally do not see a problem with the shutting down of borders in such an event. During the very early stages of the COVID panic – around December 2019/January 2020 – there was a lot of hype about some type of strange virus that was completely devastating China. What we knew was that China had created the largest quarantine in the history of mankind, men with submachine guns and hazmat suits were patrolling the streets, and numerous other videos were surfacing in corners of the web showing people being boarded up into trucks after sneezing/coughing/being diagnosed as sick/etc.

Nobody really knew what was going on, but by all reports it looked bad. At that point, the USA still was permitting flights in and out of China, however. I'm of the mind that this didn't make any sense. We saw all of this laid before us, yet we still were permitting them to fly in here. I personally think there needs to be a complete embargo on China to begin with – why are we doing any form of business whatsoever with our enemies? – so admittedly, I may be a bit biased here.

I do not believe that there would have been anything wrong committed by shutting down our borders to such. On a smaller scale though, do the ethics change? I don't think so. In order to remain consistent, I don't believe that you can have one set of ethics for the national government and an entirely different set of ethics for the local government. Size doesn't change morality. Might does not necessarily make right. So I don't really see a problem with a small local government denying access to those who aren't citizens of that region *in such a case.*

What about property owners though? What about American citizens who were currently abroad in China at the time? Do we still let them back in? I would say yes. Even within the example of our small, 17,500 people strong community, I still say yes. If somebody is a citizen, let them in. They are one of our own, and we take care of our own. To deny them access is to do them wrong. So for full-time residents, I don't see a problem here.

What about for those who are Chinese citizens who own American property? In our small-town example, what about northerners who don't reside here permanently, but instead own vacation property where we are at? Do we let them in?

Once more, if they are property owners, I think we do indeed let them in. To deny somebody access to their own property is a form of theft, that I don't think should be tolerated. Even if that person who owns such isn't a full-time citizen of that region.

What about those who don't own any property within the region? Do we let them in? I don't think so. They don't have any rightful claim to our location, they aren't part of our home, and as such they don't have any right to be here after the set border closure date. They will be turned away, and by armed force if need be.

Alright, but what do we do about the family members and friends who undoubtedly are going to try to get in as well? What about the college students who are away at the time? In such a case, if an individual – such as a child – is under the care of a current resident, I say let them in. They are still a citizen of the region, they were just away prior to the border closure date. What about other family? If we're talking about a grandparent that did indeed live within the community with their children, but was away before the closure date, I say let them in. They lived there before, and they should still be able to.

What about friends and extended family – those who are not citizens of the region, own no property within the region, but have (maybe) received an invite from citizens within our borders to stay with them to "ride this thing out". Do we permit them within the boundaries? I don't see why we should. If they've missed the border closure date, they do not get in. Sorry. No exceptions.

What about circumstances where elderly parents in our community were living independently within our boundaries but were receiving a lot of outside help from a child in a neighboring community. This could very easily be the case in a situation where you have nursing homes or assisted living communities present. Perhaps it's vice versa where a resident would regularly travel to a nearby town to care for his elderly mother. What do we do then?

I believe the fairest thing to do in such an event is to give a public warning before the border closure, telling residents what is about to happen, and to make arrangements for their loved ones as soon as possible. If that requires bringing them back to the house, then they should do so as quickly as possible. If that means leaving the boundaries to not return, they should also do so as quickly as possible. Keep in mind that such a stance also implies that those who are residents who decide to leave the community after the border closure date do so with the understanding that they will not be permitted to return afterwards – regardless of what property they own there. A week's notice should be a very practical and lenient amount of time to permit residents to make as many arrangements as they need to in order to avoid family problems.

By contacting all of the residents of a locale (perhaps through an emergency text message system?) everybody who owned property within the location could be notified that withing seven days all access was going to be blocked.

How are supplies to get into the blocked off location? This would be the tricky part. Individual and independent farmers seem to no longer exist within the United States, and it seems that this is likely to be the chink in the armor here. Up until about a hundred years ago, there were millions of farmers throughout the United States. Food was grown and sold locally. While there most certainly has been a resurgence of such throughout the past 20 years, we're still nowhere near where we once were in relation to the number of farmers.

Food now travels farther from farm to plate than it ever has before, and this requires long-distance trucking and nightmarish logistics. For this "castle community" policy to work, residents need to be ensured that they will not only have enough food and water, but that they will have the medicine and healthcare access that they are going to need as well. The dialysis patient that has to receive treatment just outside of the city borders is thus going to have a problem.

This is yet another fantastic reason why Americans need to be encouraged to keep a proper supply of emergency food and other goods on hand at all times. We now live in a world of EMPs, bioterrorist attacks, and potential pandemics that can absolutely bring the US to its knees. If we know such, why do we continue to live as if nothing bad will ever happen? Why not do something to prepare for such eventualities? People save money for retirement, knowing that at some point in the future they'll no longer be able to work, why not do the same for food?

The community that pushes for its citizens to be independent and disaster ready will be much more "disaster proof" than the community that does not. Like a castle preparing to be put under siege, this helps to enable the refuge dwellers the ability to last as long as possible based off of what is already within the castle's walls. To get more supplies in, the best bet is to probably have a system of unloading/loading locations scattered about the perimeter. Armed forces will man each "port" ensuring that supplies are not stolen in much the same way that the Coast Guard protects American ports. Buyers and sellers will then be able to trade their goods in a manner that does not bring stowaways, outsiders, and so on into the community.

Admittedly, none of this is a foolproof plan, but perhaps such will at least give you food for thought as you consider your own plan of what should be done in such a situation to protect individual rights while simultaneously protecting a community against a pandemic.

19

Mandatory Masking

"Those who are willing to surrender their freedom for security have always demanded that if they give up their full freedom it should also be taken from those not prepared to do so." – FA Hayek[1]

Polio, though not completely eradicated from the world, is incredibly close to being so. It's only been within the past fifty years that people have quit getting polio vaccinations. Why? Because on a population level, the risk well outweighed the reward.

With mass polio vaccination programs, there are going to be people who will actually develop polio, and as a result, mass vaccinations have ceased for this particular infectious agent. I wonder if the same principle doesn't apply to COVID-19. Is mass masking doing more harm than good? Are we going to end up with patients who DO develop lung infections, aneurysms, eye damage, kidney damage, and the like as a result of these mass maskings?

Why did I notice an average 20mmHg increase in my patients' blood pressures when they were wearing a mask? This is anecdotal evidence, to be sure, but it was a very common occurrence. Others had similar fears.

Guy Crittenden, the former editor of *HazMat Management,* a popular trade magazine for those involved in hazmat occupations had this to say: "the kinds of masks people are wearing were never designed to be worn for long periods and doing so is very harmful." He further added that operating rooms actually pump extra oxygen into the rooms in order to compensate for the reduction in oxygen flow that is commonplace with mask wearing.[2]

If one is truly concerned about the risk of infection, I believe that the best option is *for that particular person* to invest in and wear a N95 or N99 mask. Those are the *only* masks that are going to actually stop coronavirus. Not a bandana, not a scarf, not a T-shirt, not a cloth mask, not a surgical mask. And if such a person IS wearing a N95 or N99 mask, then there is no reason for anybody else around them to wear a mask. The concerned person is already protected! 95-99% of all airborne virus particles will be filtered out by their mask!

"What about asymptomatic spreaders though?"

I really don't see how this changes anything. If someone is still concerned about COVID-19, their choice to wear a N95 or N99 is still the best bet. To force everyone in the room to wear a surgical mask that is designed to stop droplets such as blood, vomit, or spit from entering the mouth of a healthcare provider, and *not* designed to stop virus particles is truly rather pointless.

An Ulterior Motive?

There comes a point where one has to ask whether or not there isn't some ulterior motive behind a façade when truly ridiculous rules are given. Such is the case when one looks at Maine's Governor Janet Mills decreeing in August of 2020 that restaurant staff must wear an anti-COVID cone that can only be described as a dog cone in order to prevent staff from having their breath directed down towards customers.

According to the decree, "front-of-house staff in restaurants who choose to wear face shields must now wear them upside down so that they are attached to the collar instead of the forehead, so that their breath is directed up, not down."[3]

The act of mandatory masking throughout 2020 and 2021 reached a point of ridiculousness that can best be characterized as the criminalization of the innocent. In many school districts, failing to wear a mask now counts as a dress code violation. Utah actually takes things a step farther in their schools. If you don't wear a mask there, you're guilty of a criminal misdemeanor.[4]

It was surprising to see the depths that people were willing to fall to in order to follow through with this tyranny. A San Diego Starbucks employee (Lenin Gutierrez. I personally find the name of Lenin fitting here.) actually denied service to a customer who didn't have a mask on in June of 2020.[5] This was big news at the time, though it may seem trite at the moment. It seems as everyone knows or has witnessed somebody get kicked out of a store or refused service because they refused to wear a mask. I personally witnessed pulmonary patients be told that they couldn't enter a building if they did not have a mask strapped across their face. Men who already had trouble breathing as it was, forced to have multiple layers of cloth/material across their face. If you've ever met anybody with COPD you can attest to the fact that it's incredibly difficult for them to breathe as it is. Now imagine what it looks like with a mask.

Furthermore, can we truly claim that we are working in the public's best interest when we ban masks that actually *do* filter out virus particles? Viruses are incredibly small, often being within .005 - .3 microns. Any material with a pore size larger than a virus is not virus-proof. In essence, it's like trying to keep mosquitoes out with a chain link fence. When CDC scientists work with dangerous viruses, they always have a respirator on, and often in the form of a gigantic bubble suit in a negative pressure room. For the lay person, such protection is likely to be impossible or unaffordable. What is available for the commercial market, however, is what is called a N95 mask. An N95 is commonly sold at hardware stores for those who are working with insulation, paint, dust, or the like. The pore sizes on such a mask are able to filter out 95% of airborne particulates. For those who want even further protection, there are N99 masks available on the market as well, which filter out 99% of airborne particulates. Both N95 and N99 masks *do* filter out viruses. A cloth mask, or even a surgical mask, do not.

The pore sizes in surgical masks are about 30 times larger than the average COVID virus. Cotton masks are even worse. They have pore sizes that are *hundreds* of times larger than COVID-19. The esteemed Dr. Fauci even parroted this common knowledge at the beginning of 2020 (February 17) when he said during an interview with USA Today, "If you look at the masks that you buy in a drug store, the leakage around that doesn't do much to protect you...Now, in the United States, there is absolutely no reason to wear a mask."[6]

Knowing this, isn't it strange that the CDC in August of 2020 announce that masks with valves do not protect people from transmitting the virus from others – in effect discouraging the use of such masks.[3] The great majority of masks on the market at the time that were N95 or N99 contained one-way valves. Those with valves were really the only option that actually did offer anybody any protection against an airborne virus.

What benefit is there in telling the public that a mask that will protect them won't protect others?

Proof of such can be seen by what happened at Fort Benning in Georgia during May of 2020. Despite mandatory masking of all military personnel, the fort allegedly experienced a COVID outbreak – most of these cases being asymptomatic. First, one has to wonder if there is truly and danger to an asymptomatic disease outbreak. Second, one has to wonder if the masks are working at all. Hawaii was another great example of the masks not working. Despite having near universal mask compliance since April of 2020 and some of the most severe lockdown rules throughout the US, by August, Hawaii had experienced nearly a 700% increase in cases over the past 30 days prior.[7]

So what gives? Why enforce a ruling that clearly doesn't work? I believe that Ayn Rand gave the best answer to such a question:

"When men feel that strongly about an issue, yet refuse to name it, when they fight savagely for some seemingly incoherent, unintelligible goal – one may be sure that their actual goal would not stand public identification."[8]

What this actual goal was, I'll leave to the reader to decide. Thankfully, however, the entire world didn't cave to such blatant stupidity. Henning Bundgaard, the chief physician at Denmark's Righospitale had this to say: "All these countries recommending face masks haven't made their decisions based on new studies." Other experts seemed to agree.

Coen Berends, the spokesman for the National Institute of Public Health and the Environment, said this: "Face masks in public places are not necessary, based on all the current evidence." Tamara van Ark, the Medical Care Minister of Denmark, said," From a medical point of view, there is no evidence of a medical effect of wearing face masks, so we decided not to impose a national obligation. Sweden's top infectious disease expert, Anders Tegnell, said, "With numbers diminishing very quickly in Sweden, we see no point in wearing a face mask in Sweden, not even on public transport."

Even the US CDC agreed with the rest of the world on this subject before the politicization of the virus reached full tilt. On February 27, 2020, the CDC posted on Twitter that they did not recommend the use of masks to protect against COVID, instead saying that washing hands and staying home when sick were more useful actions.[9]

Anders Tengell of Sweden had more to say on the issue. "It is very dangerous to believe face masks would change the game when it comes to COVID-19." He went on to say, "The findings that have been produced through face masks are astonishingly weak, even though many people around the world wear them...Countries such as Spain and Belgium have made their populations wear mask, but their infection numbers have still risen."[10]

It's interesting to note that Muslim countries faced sky-high diagnoses rates as well. Within Sharia law, women must wear a hijab to cover their face from men. If they show their face, then they can be subjected to flogging, beating, or even potentially execution. Despite an entire culture where 50% of the populace has worn a cloth face covering for the greater majority of their adult life, they *still* had high rates. So if cloth masks are helping, why didn't it help Islamic nations?

So what was the end culprit here? Why did the entire world suddenly agree simultaneously that the entire globe needed to be masked? Once more, let the reader draw their own conclusions.

Even the CDC eventually – though albeit somewhat accidentally – admitted that the masks that they had been proponents of for so long actually may have not worked as well as they claimed they did. During September of 2020 – after terrible wildfires absolutely ravaged the state of California – the CDC came out and told people that they could not expect cloth masks to protect them from the severely poor air quality, saying that smoke particulates are actually too small to be stopped by a cloth mask.

A smoke particle is typically anywhere between 0.4 to 0.7 microns in size. COVID-19 is 0.12 microns in size – about a fourth of the size of a smoke particle.[11]

So while cloth masks are touted as being ineffective for smoke – a relatively larger particle – the public was told that they were perfectly safe for those who were concerned about coronavirus.

September of 2020 was a big month for the CDC. It was on September 11's Morbidity and Mortality Weekly Report that it was shown that 85% of those who had contracted COVID during July either always wore a mask when out in public or often wore one the two weeks prior to their infection. How could this happen? If the masks are everything that they were flouted by the government to be, this shouldn't even be possible! This MMWR went on to show that over 70% of those infected reported always wearing masks. Now here's the real kicker: only *3.9%* of those testing positive for COVID reported *never* wearing a mask.[12]

How could anybody look at this data and come to the conclusion that one still needs to wear a mask? This data clearly shows that *not* wearing a mask is a much safer alternative than wearing one. It makes one wonder if there isn't a more sinister purpose behind the mandatory masking that the world saw throughout 2020.

This author has a number of hypothesis why this may be the case. Chief among these would be the research that proves that those who regularly wear cloth masks actually *increase* their chances of getting a lung infection.[13] Breathing in your own carbon dioxide and mouth bacteria all day long doesn't seem to actually be beneficial to anybody. Combine that with the fact that most peoples' masks are reused multiple times and you have a virtual petri dish that is being strapped to your face so that you can suck the bacteria out of it as you go about your daily basis.

I also believe that the uncomfortableness of masks plays a factor. Masks constantly move about your face as you talk, yawn, breathe, and laugh. It's because of this that you consistently have to touch and readjust it. Your fingers are arguably the dirtiest part of your body. You wouldn't ever lick a door handle to a public library, yet you likely have adjusted your mask after opening that same handle – placing those door handle germs on a mask strapped to your face. This has to have some effect in transmitting sickness.

What Should We Do Then with Forced Masking?

So as a public health professional, what can we do? What is the appropriate response to contagious disease that can be spread via air? In such a case, should government decree mandatory masking throughout its domain? Does it violate human rights, and does the government therefore have a right to make such a decree?

The answer?

Absolutely not, and those who would argue otherwise are those who simply repeat what their propaganda tells them to, in much the same manner as the sheep from *Animal Farm* who only bleat the same slogan louder and louder whenever anybody counters their dogma with facts. The constant bleating of such sheep only takes on new levels of stupidity once one remembers that there is truly no need for it.

If there is a contagious respiratory illness encircling the globe the correct response of public health and government officials is to *encourage* N95 or N99 use. Those who use either of these types of masks will effectively protect themselves from airborne illnesses and have little to nothing to fear about being in close proximity to strangers. To encourage *any* type of mask is to lie to the people, for wearing a cloth mask is absolutely zero protection, and a surgical mask is designed to protect a surgeon from getting blood or other body fluids in his mouth while he is operating and to protect the patient from getting spit inside of them – *not* for protecting either party against airborne particles.

To *force* people to wear an N95 is ludicrous and an overstepping of governmental authority. Those who choose to do so – due to the freedom bought for them at the price of the blood and lives of American patriots – are protected, and are therefore in no need for others to be forced to wear a mask that adds zero extra protection to their own self. Let man choose his risk. If man decides to risk going out in public with no mask in such a situation, so be it. If man decides to not do so by wearing a N95, then so be it.

There is zero need for any governmental authority to step in and make such a decision for them.

As Ayn Rand said, "No man can have a right to impose an unchosen obligation, an unrewarded duty or an involuntary servitude on another man. There can be no such thing as the 'right to enslave'".[14] The forcing of others to wear masks – not effective ones, mind you – but instead ones to solely virtue signal is to enforce a new form of tyranny against the public. It is to reach an age where there are those who believe that they are morally superior because they won't show their face in public. If only they would go all the way...

Furthermore, I believe that the Founding Fathers of the USA would have quite a bit to say about the concept of forced masking. If we take a look at the little read Declaration of Independence, we find that these truths are considered self-evident: that mankind is given unalienable rights by God, and among these are life, liberty, and the pursuit of happiness. Does oxygen not apply to any of these? Is it not necessary for life? Is it not therefore necessary for the other two as well?

20

Quarantine

Does a government have the right to forcibly detain an individual in the name of quarantine? If so, what are the necessary qualifications that must be established first so that we're not using such as a pretext for unlimited detainment? And speaking of time, how long is it appropriate to keep an individual locked in quarantine? Are there benefits that they deserve for going through such?

These are all some of the questions that we will seek to answer within this section, as we analyze whether or not quarantine can coincide with human rights, or if it even deserves to be a concept in the first place. The answer may surprise you.

As usual, let's start by looking at the COVID panic to see if there are lessons that we can glean from that particular period of history.

2020 and Quarantine

It was in October of 2020 that New York's Governor Cuomo decreed that all visitors to New York would have to quarantine for three days upon entering the state in order to prove that they were negative for the virus before they were "free to go about their business". Before that though, you must first show proof of a negative test. So you must have a negative test, quarantine for three more days, and then get yet another COVID test on the fourth day. If you refuse to get tested for COVID, then you must quarantine for a total of 14 days before you are "free to go about your business".[1]

Is such a mandate justified, or is it a violation of human rights? Is the act of quarantine in and of itself a violation of human rights? Should quarantine be abolished as a concept altogether? It is here that we're going to examine such questions.

For starters, we need to differentiate between quarantine and isolation. The act of quarantine is to forcibly separate somebody from others, typically due to the desire/need to protect healthy people from sick people. The act of isolation is to tell somebody that they need to stay away from others, but not to forcibly remove them. I personally believe that both of them have their place and time.

Why is this?

The Bible's Laws on Quarantine

If we look within the Old Testament, we will find some of the earliest recorded public health laws in the history of mankind. Seeing that Christian ideals were the foundation of the US Constitution and concept of inherent human rights (not to mention these were laws given by God – the fairest and most just judge that anyone will ever meet), I believe that this is an excellent place to start our analysis of what is a violation of human rights when it comes to quarantine.

Within Old Testament times there were a number of contagious illnesses that were easily spread throughout a community just as there are today. Chief of these sicknesses would be leprosy. It's interesting to note that while we typically think of the word leprosy that we think of leprosy proper – (Hansen's disease) – the skin condition where people gradually rot away and limbs and appendages fall off, but that throughout the Bible the term "leprosy" is actually used to describe a wide host of health issues. For proof of this just look at the laws regarding a house catching leprosy, where it appears that they occasionally had issues with dangerous molds growing indoors.

"When you have come into the land of Canaan, which I give you as a possession, and I put the leprous plague in a house in the land of your possession, and he who owns the house comes and tells the priest, saying, 'It seems to me that there is *some plague in the house,' then the priest shall command that they empty the house, before the priest goes* into it *to examine the plague, that all that is in the house may not be made unclean; and afterward the priest shall go in to examine the house. And he shall examine the plague; and indeed* if the plague *is on the walls of the house with ingrained streaks, greenish or reddish, which appear to be deep in the wall, then the priest shall go out of the house, to the door of the house, and shut up the house seven days.* – Leviticus 14: 34-38

If somebody from this time was suspected of having leprosy, the first thing that they had to do was to get checked out by the priest. If the priest – using a *pre-established* set of criteria for deciding what was potentially dangerous and what was not – examined the sore, boil, rash, etc. and determined that it *did* meet the criteria for being a potential danger, the probable infected man was forcibly quarantined away from the rest of the community. This was to prevent the spread of infectious disease throughout the rest of the Jewish tribes.

You can see this evidenced in the following verses:

"When a man has on the skin of his body a swelling, a scab, or a bright spot, and it becomes on the skin of his body like a leprous sore, then he shall be brought to Aaron the priest or to one of his sons the priests. The priest shall examine the sore on the skin of the body; and if the hair on the sore has turned white, and the sore appears to be deeper than the skin of his body, it is a leprous sore. Then the priest shall examine him, and pronounce him unclean.
– Leviticus 13:2-3

This is just a snippet of chapter 13 of Leviticus, where a wide range of maladies are discussed, but it will give you the idea as to how this was done in Biblical times. There was a very specific set of criteria given ahead of time for what made one unclean. There were also a very specific set of rules to be followed if one was found to be unclean. We can see that from the following:

"Now the leper on whom the sore is, his clothes shall be torn and his head bare; and he shall cover his mustache, and cry, 'Unclean! Unclean!' He shall be unclean. All the days he has the sore he shall be unclean. He is unclean, and he shall dwell alone; his dwelling shall be outside the camp.
– Leviticus 13:45-46

Specific instructions were given as to where the man was to go, how long he was to stay there, and what the requirements were for him to reenter society. Oftentimes after a set period of time the man would once more visit the priest for reexamination. If he passed the exam – the issue had stayed the same, or the issue had diminished – the man was permitted back into society. He wasn't a danger to others. If the man failed the exam – the issue had grown worse – he was either quarantined for a further period of time or banished from the community entirely. In the case of leprosy, this involved being sent to live in a leper community.

I believe that this is an appropriate course of action for infectious diseases when it comes to crafting any type of quarantine law. If an issue is discovered – if a man exhibits signs and symptoms that could most certainly be associated with a dangerous contagious illness – I don't see any problem whatsoever with asking him to isolate from others until further examinations can be made. I don't see any problem in forcible quarantine in certain situations either.

Now, we don't know this for sure, the Bible doesn't specifically state such, but it would make sense that there would be consequences if a leper tried to break this law of quarantine. Would the healthy Israelites have suffered an unclean leper who was contagious and breaking the law to have mingled freely within the camp? I imagine they had the means and wherewithal to keep lepers out by force if that was necessitated. I do not see how this is an injustice in this case.

Let's say that there was a smallpox outbreak throughout the United States. Nobody is vaccinated against such anymore, and it would be likely if such *were* to occur that it would be the result of a bioterrorist/biowarfare attack with a weaponized strain that our vaccinations would likely be ineffective against in the first place. The pox is ravaging the United States, having popped up in multiple areas simultaneously, and is spreading like wildfire. Early signs and symptoms include a fever, malaise, and a very distinctive rash developing along the chest and limbs.

If a man shows up to a doctor's clinic exhibiting all of those signs and symptoms in such a situation, I see no issue whatsoever in quarantining him. To not do so is to leave an infectious person out in society where he will continue to spread the illness to others. Seeing that this is going to be a deadly disease, his being in society will lead to people dying due to smallpox.

As such, it is justified to quarantine this man. This was the response that was taken throughout the Old Testament, and if it was just then, it is just now. God doesn't change. He is immutable.

"Prevention" Can Soon Prove to Be Tyranny

In contrast, would it be morally justifiable to forcibly quarantine a man who had no signs or symptoms, felt absolutely fine, and to all appearances was as healthy as could be? I would argue no. To do so in this case would be to imprison somebody for absolutely no reason other than fear. If we let this type of imprisonment become public policy, it will soon spawn a host of further abuses of power as people throughout the country will be kidnapped and thrown into cells against their will with a laundry list of potential reasons being given as to why they are unsafe to be in society.

Think of the implications of imprisoning the healthy. Any personal vendetta by a politician, police officer, or even an angry neighbor could be instantly fulfilled. All that would need to be done is to make a report and send people to the address of where the intended victim could be found, giving something along the lines of saying that they had been acting ill of late and needed to be quarantined.

At this point the person would be arrested by men in hazmat suits with rifles, he would be chained, thrown into a vehicle (where true infected may have sat moments prior), and then hauled away to a quarantine/prison facility for an indefinite period of time. While in this facility, this man may be placed in a cell where a truly ill person had been placed a day before. He may be placed in a cell with several other people – even those who are truly ill. His family may be deprived of his protection, his provision, and his comfort as well during this trying time. During his stay, the man may even be subjected to medical treatments and testing that he does not want.

Perhaps the doctors on site will force the man to several blood tests, anal swab, nasal swabs, or even mandate a blood transfusion, vaccination, or other medical procedure. All against this man's will.

These are all possibilities when we permit the forcible quarantining of the healthy. To my knowledge, this was never done throughout the Old Testament. Those who slept with a woman with an abnormal discharge of blood were considered unclean for a number of days after having sex (Leviticus 15:19-24), but this was somebody who had just had sex with someone who may have had a contagious disease. There were times when people were labeled unclean if they had ejaculated (Leviticus 15:16), started their period (Leviticus 15:19), or had a wound (Leviticus 15:1-12), but this doesn't seem to have resulted in forced quarantine in these situations, but instead in being unable to access the temple. Witness the following verses:

'If a woman has a discharge, and *the discharge from her body is blood, she shall be set apart seven days; and whoever touches her shall be unclean until evening.*

Everything that she lies on during her impurity shall be unclean; also everything that she sits on shall be unclean. Whoever touches her bed shall wash his cloths and bathe in water, and be unclean until evening. And whoever touches anything that she sat on shall wash his clothes and bathe in water, and be unclean until evening. If anything is on her bed or on anything on which she sits, when he touches it, he shall be unclean until evening. And if any man lies with her at all, so that her impurity is on him, he shall be unclean seven days; and every bed on which he lies shall be unclean.
– Leviticus 15:19-24

This seems to indicate that the woman with a discharge, though unclean, was still permitted to live in her house. She was unclean, but she was still healthy. No forcible quarantine seems to have taken place. After all, there's explicit mention on what to do if her husband has sex with her during this time. If she was forcibly quarantined, I don't see how this would have been possible.

Overall, I think it's fair to say that I don't see any evidence of anybody other than those with signs or symptoms of disease that were ever forcibly quarantined within the Bible, and I believe that we should follow the same precautions today. And this is what I mean by that: if somebody is exhibiting signs or symptoms of an incredibly dangerous and deadly contagious disease, only then should we consider the act of quarantine. We do not quarantine the healthy. Nor do we go out looking for "the asymptomatic".

The next question may be, "Well, how do we know who the healthy are? What if somebody is an asymptomatic spreader of the illness? Don't we have a right to know who such people are?"

I would give an unequivocal 'no' as the answer here. If you believe that you have the right to know the status of every single person around you, you are opening the door for a wide number of tyrannies to creep through. You are in effect deeming that nobody around you has the right to privacy, that your fear entitles you to the violation of others' human rights, and that *you* have the right to *force* medical procedures on others, among other things. If we permit this train of logic to flourish, we once more end up in a world where mandatory vaccinations, mandatory sterilizations, mandatory medical procedures, and other forms of medical tyranny are not only permitted but are widely supported as well.

This is opening the door for a nightmare.

When you begin to focus on prevention of illness, it is very easy to take things to an extreme that is unjustified. John Stuart Mill illustrated this in his book *On Liberty*. He said, "The preventive function of government, however, is far more liable to be abused, to the prejudice of liberty, than the punitory function; for there is hardly any part of the legitimate freedom of action of a human being which would not admit of being represented, and fairly too, as increasing the facilities for some form or other of delinquency."[2]

The same has been done before with the concept of crime prevention. While I most certainly support peoples' decisions to lock their doors when they go out, to keep their blinds shut at night, to not leave valuables in sight in their vehicles while they go out – all valid means of preventing criminals from being criminals – if you allow prevention to become the sole focus of legislation, you quickly end up in a *Minority Report* type of situation.

You end up in a world where pre-crime exists. Where the *probability* that you would commit a crime is enough to incriminate and punish you. This is a world where an algorithm could predict that you were 88% likely to engage in an anti-government act (e.g. blogging about tyranny), and the state would then believe that they were justified in throwing you into prison for 15 years. You hadn't *done* anything that was a crime. You were just *likely* to. At least, according to the metrics and algorithms used by the state.

We can very easily end up in the same set of world with public health if we allow the concept of prevention to be taken too far. If we decide upon a policy of preventing every case at all costs, then we will believe that we are justified in perpetuating medical tyranny upon a populace. While prevention is most certainly worthwhile and a worthy endeavor up to an extent, it can easily be taken too far.

Keep in mind that throughout the Old Testament leprosy was a *constant* threat. It never disappeared. Despite this, you never saw any mandates made where once a month every Israelite was required to be given a complete exam by the priest. Never once was this even suggested. It was only required for those with signs and symptoms. If we do *that* – if we get those people to understand that they need to see a doctor – then we are doing what we can to engage in prevention without violating human rights.

We can then take appropriate measures that are further preventative acts if we discover that the man does indeed have the contagious and deadly illness that we're afraid of. This *is* doing something. It's not being idle and sitting on our hands as things play their natural course to completion. But it's a way to do something without becoming a monster in the process. If somebody doesn't like this – if they believe that such a stance only places them at risk – then may I recommend moving to an area where you feel safer. Perhaps Australia, France, England, or some other nation with draconian health laws is more up your alley. America doesn't seem to be a good fit for you.

Which Diseases Do We Quarantine Against?

So the next question that we must ask is this: what illnesses is quarantine justified for? While nobody will see any problem with quarantining somebody with Ebola, smallpox, or bubonic plague, what about illnesses such as seasonal flu? Flu kills people, does it not? Is this something that we thus need to have mandatory quarantine for?

Here are my thoughts: we've already created a classification for infectious agents regarding how dangerous they are. This is the basis for the various levels (or tiers) of biological agent labs that we have throughout the world. At the very top (Level 1), are the most dangerous infectious agents in the world. It's here that we find plague, smallpox, Q fever, and others. Level 2 labs are for dangerous agents that are slightly less dangerous than Level 1. And Level 3 is for even less dangerous agents.

If we've *already* created a tier system, why reinvent the wheel? We've never considered seasonal flu as a Level 1 agent. So why start so – with all the implications of such – now? While there could most certainly be an argument made for a novel form of pandemic influenza that was leaving mounds of corpses in its wake, this would have to be *factually proven*. There would need to be definitive numbers of a mass death situation. This couldn't be a situation akin to the 2020 COVID scam where the numbers were made up, the testing procedures were incredibly sensitive to bump up the numbers, and where 99.7% of those infected lived after the fact. This would have to be a *true* pandemic influenza that was a harbinger of death in order to be considered.

If this new pandemic influenza was *justly* classified as a Level 1 biological agent, *then* I believe that we would be justified in engaging in appropriate quarantine procedures *amongst those who were exhibiting signs and symptoms.*

Practically, I don't believe that it is proper to send out crews of armed men in hazmat suits to search through a population to see who is sick and who is not by going door to door. Such is an invasion of privacy, would be a massive waste of resources, and would quickly lead to government-mandated kidnapping (amongst other evils). The best option would be via self-reporting. This would be accomplished by the sick visiting a doctor, calling a doctor, or willfully notifying somebody else that they were indeed sick.

If any illness is bad enough, the sick may not even be able to get out of bed. If such is the case, a family member may have to pick up the slack for them, doing what they can to ensure that their family member is going to receive the care that they need (while keeping themselves safe in the process). If the only way that a family member can do this is by calling the doctor to put in a notification, then so be it.

Throughout the Black Death, there were numerous families who were left in a state of helplessness as a family member got sick with the plague. Examples of such are detailed again and again throughout Daniel Defoe's *Journal of the Plague Year.* When a mother became sick, often the only thing that family members could do was seal off the door and wait. Nobody knew that it was fleas that were carrying the disease from person to person. All they knew was that exposure to the sick would virtually always result in your becoming mortally ill as well.

Ingenuity was often resorted to in order to find novel ways of ensuring that the ill had access to food and water, but the family members would often report the illness to authorities directly or indirectly by putting a sign on their front door. This is a form of notification that I see no problem with. If someone is instructed to put a piece of orange paper on their front door should there be a Level 1 infected within the household, this is an easy way to inform others that there *are* sick inside, that they are to be avoided, and that they can be accounted for as well. This is likely to be one of the best ways to handle mass amounts of sick people that would otherwise easily overwhelm the medical infrastructure of a nation.

To come to the conclusion of the matter, quarantine does need to exist as both a concept and a policy (it was used within the Bible), but we have to be very vigilant that we keep it within its proper domains and that we do not engage in it with minimal justification.

21

Vaccine Scheduling

"Casting lots causes contentions to cease, and keeps the mighty apart." – Proverbs 18:18, NKJV

Who deserves vaccines first? Such can potentially be a problematic conundrum for authorities when a pandemic is raging. And the answer to such a question does seem to depend on a variety of factors – particularly around the characteristics of the disease itself.

For example, let's assume that there is a novel variant of flu circling the earth much like the Spanish flu of 1918. This strain isn't picky. It doesn't matter if one is male or female, black or white, young or old. It doesn't differentiate. The death rate is high, it's incredibly contagious, and people across the planet are dying from it in droves. Cemeteries are having a hard time keeping up with the workload as are funeral directors. Mass graves are the current topic in the media, and as unpleasant as it sounds, it *does* seem as if that's where things are going to go next. But then, a miracle occurs. A vaccine is discovered. Production of it is slow at first, as should be expected, as facilities gear up their factories and laboratories for the production of as much of the vaccine as they can.

And the vaccine works great as well. There are no side effects of significant consequence, and the vaccine is 98%

effective. Much like smallpox or polio, if you get the vaccine, you don't have to worry about getting the disease.

In such a situation, the US may only be able to create 100,000 vaccines in the first batch. How do you decide who gets those? How do you decide who gets the following batches? The decision of such is in essence determining whose life is more important than others. In such a scenario, the denial of a vaccine to one in favor of another is to throw another straggler off of the lifeboat, telling them to take their chances out in the open water.

It goes without a doubt that the first to get the vaccine are going to be those who work within government, both in the form of politicians and in soldiers. I believe that this is to be expected. I suppose it's one of the perks of the job. Most would likely argue that healthcare workers should be the next in line. Without those to work in healthcare, the entire healthcare system falls apart. Heart attacks, strokes, gunshot wounds, and other common maladies do not stop just because a pandemic has started. There will still be a need for doctors, nurses, phlebotomists, and others to work on those issues. However, with the addition of a global pandemic the need for healthcare workers will increase exponentially. This will be due to the fact that not only will there be an exponential increase in the amount of sickness and death across the world, but also due to there being a large number of healthcare workers who become sick and/or die from the illness as well. Others will retire, quit, or simply refuse to show up to work (can you blame them?). As a result of all of these factors combined, hospitals and clinics will be incredibly short staffed to deal with an already dangerous and terrible situation.

Perchance healthcare workers are not at the front of the line for such a vaccine there is a very real probability that they could collectivize and threaten to quit; refusing to treat patients unless they were taken care of first. The argument would run that without a vaccine, their care for flu patients would be nothing more than a game of Russian roulette – a suicide game. Millions would die without those healthcare workers, and during such a time, politicians will not have the ability to risk the chance of more healthcare workers leaving in droves or refusing to show up to work. Quite simply, they would *have* to give in to the demands of the healthcare workers. Those within the hospital system would hold an enormous amount of power in this respect, and it is unlikely there would be a politician stupid enough to risk playing such a game.

While I could potentially see some politicians across the globe enacting "emergency power" laws mandating that healthcare workers show up to work and treat patients regardless of whether or not they as workers had actually received the vaccine, as a whole, I don't think that such would be a common procedure.

So after politicians, after soldiers, after healthcare workers, how do you decide who comes next? What is the best course of action for the greater part of the American public? Public health authorities have to be incredibly careful with what their decision is, because if they do not choose correctly (and I do believe that there is only one correct choice here), there is going to be violence. If the correct decision is not made, there will be widescale rioting, looting, killing of those who give/have gotten the vaccine, and theft of the remaining amounts of vaccine.

Given the nature of our hypothetical flu strain, I would argue that the best option, the *only* one that will minimize the risk of violence is to utilize a lottery system much akin to that used in Matt Damon's *Contagion*. A very publicized lottery needs to be put in place where the public has as much trust as possible in the process. There needs to be as close to zero doubt as possible that the lottery wasn't rigged. If possible, it needs to be shown that all outcomes of the lottery are of equal probability. As such, any form of computerized system should not even be considered.

The lottery needs to be comprised of something where the internal workings are as visible as possible. As such, I truly believe that a bingo hall style ball spinner is likely one of the best ways to go. The public has little reason to believe that any of the balls have been rigged, and I can't foresee a way that one could rig a bingo ball to increase its chance of going first. Potentially, that could be accomplished by making one weigh more than the others, but the idea of such being a possibility could be eliminated by individually weighing each ball publicly beforehand on a scale.

The best method to determine what the bingo balls are going to say is most likely to be by going by either birth date or alphabetical by last name. For birth date, that may entail saying everyone born on a particular day, in a particular week, or a particular month. Alphabetically by last name is most certainly an option as well. Social security numbers could not be used as that would completely leave out the entire Amish community and potentially many others who have rejected social security on religious principles. Going by state would only develop animosity between the states. Perchance California or New York were chosen as the first states to receive immunity – while this would most certainly be easier logistically speaking; to ship all of the vaccines to one state and coordinate within that one region rather than across the entire nation – such an action would infuriate the greater part of America that views both of these states as antithetical to American principles.

Having the lottery system choose by age group would most likely lead to animosity as well. Perchance older people between 80-85 were chosen as the first recipients there would likely be strikes and walk offs of workers across the nation (particularly healthcare workers who would like to see their spouses and children vaccinated), violence against that particular age group, and most certainly public outrage against such a group as well. The arguments would run along the lines of that age group having already lived a full life and depending upon the care of others. It would be argued as well that they would be immunized only to die a year later, and that we would be leaving the country to a decrepit nursing home.

If children were immunized first – say ages 0-5 – there wouldn't be as much of a public outrage as it would be political suicide to fight against infants and children, but the argument would be raised that it does no good to leave a bunch of children on the earth alone. The only age grouping that would be tolerated as a first choice would be those between 15 – 55 most likely.

However, all of this could be avoided by simply going by birth or alphabetical by last name. It would be important to make the distinction that prisoners and illegal aliens should *not* be included in the lottery. This would be a political and contentious issue that many would disagree with during the time frame that such an action was needed, but I will make the case that to include either of these groups into the lottery would be immoral and undesirable.

To begin with, if prisoners are included in the lottery there will be public outrage, and rightfully so. Should murderers, rapists, drug dealers, and pedophiles have access to a vaccine to such a disease before responsible citizens who contribute to society? I would argue no. Many of those within prisons are there because of having been involved in heinous acts. There are most certainly political prisoners as well – 2020 made a host of them, even in the United States – but there can be no distinctions made for anybody within the prison system. Those with freedom need to come first. Consider such part of the cost of being a criminal.

I don't believe that illegal immigrants even deserve much time for discussion. The term 'illegal' should be all anybody needs to hear to formulate their opinion on such a subject. Is it right for those who put money into a system to have to pay for the freeloader? Illegal immigrants have no place within a nation, and by no means should be given preference for such a vaccine over those who are actually citizens.

Only after the rest of the population as a whole has been vaccinated from this deadly disease do you turn your attention to the prisons. Such, I believe, is the only just way to proceed here.

While there are always going to be arguments made regardless of which decision is made in such a sticky situation, I truly believe that the vaccine lottery in the manner described above is the most fair way to proceed, and the only method that won't cause public outrage.

22

Curfews

Though a subject that I initially believed no rational human being would vouch for as a form of infection control, 2020 proved that there are those out there within the realm of government who will argue (against reason) otherwise. As such, I feel that it is my duty to address even this subject, to show that there must be reason and human rights considered when such a subject is discussed.

The stated reason for a curfew is that it prevents infection by decreasing the number of events a person has the opportunity to frequent, where they may in turn be exposed to or expose others to disease. It was argued that parties and bars in particular were dangerous to the public health because people gathered at both of these situations en masse and did not follow proper "safety" protocols.

This, despite the fact, that people were at work with potentially hundreds of others throughout the hours prior. This, despite the fact, that no virus or bacteria is more infectious at night. Parasites may indeed be more active at nighttime, but the coming of 10PM does not signal COVID-19 to come out of the shadows to infect people at will.

Creation of a curfew is a drastic step in the murder of human freedom. It is a very visible example of being placed under the thumb of a nanny state where grown adults are once more treated under the rules of an unruly adolescent. As if they are naughty children who must be taught a lesson by those who are inherently wiser and more virtuous than the citizens who elected them to their position in the first place.

Curfews are typically the creation of a martial law type scenario with the hopes of curtailing nighttime engagements by the enemy within a "pacified" area. This type of tool being used as a public health policy needs to be dismissed outright. People will easily see the parallel between being placed under martial law and their current situation (which is truly one and the same) if a public health official gives the ruling of a curfew.

Whether that be in the form of telling people that they can't be out at a certain time of night or telling a business owner that he can't stay open for business at what hours he prefers – either option is a gross overstepping of authority by government officials that they have no right to propose or enforce. So while this is most certainly a shorter chapter, I don't believe it needs to be any longer. Any form of curfew is not only illogical as a source of disease prevention, but an inherent violation of human rights as well.

23

The "Right" To Not Get Sick

One phrase that was flaunted throughout 2020 – 2021 was that one did not have the *right* to go about infecting others. Such was the basic premise behind mandatory masking, the talk of forced vaccinations, lockdowns, social distancing, curfews, vaccine ID cards, and the entire gamut of human rights violations that we have seen throughout this time.

But let's examine such a foundation further, shall we? Does one truly not have the right to infect somebody else? On the surface, I would agree with the question. If one has a container of smallpox that they've stolen from a lab in China, they do not have the right to disseminate that disease to infect others. Should a gay man be diagnosed with AIDS, he does not have the right to go about willfully and purposefully infecting others. Should a child have an active case of mumps – and his parents know it - , he does not have the right to go to school to purposefully spread it to classmates whom he does not like.

Nobody is arguing with the point that one does not have the right to *purposefully* infect somebody else with some type of disease or illness. However, with COVID-19, that wasn't ever really the issue. When politicians used the excuse that you didn't have the right to get somebody else sick, it truly was nothing more than a thinly veiled excuse for them to justify passing whatever arbitrary decrees they had pop into their head for that particular day. The depressing part about this though is that there were plenty of Americans out there – the most free people group on the planet – who were so poorly versed in the subjects of freedom, the Constitution, the Bill of Rights, and Americanism that they swallowed this poorly crafted logic hook, line, and sinker.

What was *really* being touted was that one had the "right" to not get sick. Such is not a right of man, has never been a right, and will never be a right on earth. To declare that one has the right to not get sick is to declare that one has the right to force everybody else that they come into contact with to live in a plastic bubble – that way they'll never risk airborne germs, droplets, or skin-to-skin contact that could get the "victim" sick. To declare that one has the "right" to not get sick is to declare that others must clean everything that the declarer may come in contact with using a cleaning agent before such a person ever gets there in the first place. To declare that one has the "right" to not get sick is to declare that one has the right to live in an absolutely sterile environment and that others must provide it for them.

This is nonsense to the extreme, and it deserves to be resisted.

Ayn Rand said it best when she said, "Any alleged 'right' of one man, which necessitates the violation of the rights of another, is not and cannot be a right."[1] She also said, "Just as in the material realm the plundering of a country's wealth is accomplished by inflating the currency – so today one may witness the process of inflation being applied to the realm of rights. The process entails such a growth of newly promulgated "rights" that people do not notice the fact that the meaning of the concept is being reserved. Just as bad money drives out good money, so these 'printing-press rights' negate authentic rights."[2]

Did we not witness this first-hand? Was it not the creation of the "right" to not get sick that quickly led to the abolishing of the right to free speech, to assemble, to defend oneself, to own property, and a host of other *God*-given rights?

By claiming that one has the right to a sterile environment (what declaring one has the right to not get sick truly means) is to declare that others are to become their personal maids and butlers; to declare that they are enslaving all of those around them, and that if those to-be slaves *don't* comply, they are to be criticized both privately and publicly. Yet it's not only to argue for criticism of the non-compliant, but also for the criminal prosecution of such as well.

There was a further twist to the "right" to not get sick throughout the COVID situation, however. Underlying the idea that one does not have the "right" to not infect somebody else was the assumption that every other person on the planet must be diseased. It was to assume that others were lepers and therefore they must be treated as such. When *all* are treated as lepers, even when they are most certainly not so, humanity quickly degrades in its reactions with itself. The very thought of human decency quickly goes right out the window, and the door is opened for the introduction of a host of demeaning and criminal actions which would have never even been thought possible beforehand.

I myself witnessed people literally screaming at others because they were standing what was deemed "too close" to them. I've witnessed people hold out their outstretched arms - as if they're directing traffic - in order to tell others that "that's far enough, ma'am. I don't want you standing any closer to me." I've witnessed arguments. You've undoubtedly seen the same, if not worse.

History has proven over and over again that when you encourage the dehumanization of others in such a way, terror soon follows. All those who argue for the right to not get sick should understand that these terrors are indeed what they are arguing for.

24

Silencing Criticism

This, then is the appropriate region of human liberty. It comprises, first, the inward domain of consciousness; demanding liberty of conscience, in the most comprehensive sense; liberty of thought and feeling; absolute freedom of opinion and sentiment on all subjects, practical or speculative, scientific, moral, or theological. –
John Stuart Mill, On Liberty[1]

"…Liberty of Thought: from which it is impossible to separate the cognate liberty of speaking and of writing." –
John Stuart Mill, On Liberty[2]

"Facts and theories must thus become no less the object of an official doctrine than views about values. And the whole apparatus for spreading knowledge – the schools and the press, radio and motion picture – will be used exclusively to spread those views which, whether true or false, will strengthen the belief in the rightness of the decisions taken by the authority; and all information that might cause doubt or hesitation will be withheld. The probable effect on the people's loyalty to the system becomes the only criterion for deciding whether a particular piece of information is to be published or suppressed." – FA Hayek[3]

Sad it is to think that America has come to the place where there truly needs to be a discussion about the ethics of silencing those who disagree with you when it comes to public health advice. Free speech, despite being a

Constitutionally-protected right, lost many proponents throughout the span of 365 days.

Imagine, if you will, that you went to the doctor for a routine physical. You really don't have anything of note to report to the doctor, but you get a physical every year as it is, and so, there you are. It's while you are there that the doctor, fresh out of medical school, states that the occasional runny nose that you get is likely due to a tapeworm infestation, and therefore, you need to quickly take a gigantic course of anti-tapeworm medicines. You're shocked, and a bit incredulous towards the doctor. You've had an occasional runny nose for years, after all, as did your father and your grandmother. It just seems to be one of those things that runs in your family. As the young doctor proceeds to tell you about the medication that he's prescribing for you, he begins to tell you the long list of side effects that the medication can have.

You're rather uncomfortable with the whole experience, and though you really think that the young doctor is out of his mind, he's now sowed seeds of doubt and fear into your mind, and so you would like to get some reassurance on the matter. You tell him thanks, but you'd like to get a second opinion first. Then in response, the doctor puts you on a patient blacklist (for the sake of argument, let's pretend there is such a thing), that makes it so no other doctor in the region will see you. You disagreed with his opinion – having good reasons to do so – and in return the doctor made it so you couldn't disagree with you in any way or shape whatsoever.

Sounds ridiculous, does it not?

Well, welcome to the beginning of the '20s, with COVID being the tapeworm infestation.

Throughout this time if a doctor, politician, or anybody said anything against the prevailing anthem regarding COVID-19 they were almost immediately silenced via a number of ways. It grew to the point that it was very clear that there was an agenda of sorts that was gracefully swimming by underneath the turbulent waves of what the greater part of the populace saw.

President Donald Trump at one point publicly stated that hydroxychloroquine seemed to show promising results in treating those with COVID. Several doctors even reported that they had seen 100% recovery rates utilizing such treatment. In response, the mainstream media (MSM) demonized HCQ and anyone who would be "stupid" enough to prescribe it. Both pharmacies and hospital systems throughout the country actually forbid their pharmacists to fill the order for the medicine or forbid their doctors to prescribe such. Several states actually threatened to revoke the medical license of doctors who prescribed HCQ to their patients.[4]

Videos posted on YouTube talking about COVID-19 that didn't align with what the MSM was touting were quickly pulled down. Facebook, Instagram, and Twitter quickly sent their fact checkers to go through posts that didn't comply with the MSM agenda regarding COVID. Any opposing voices were silenced as quickly as possible. Even scientific studies that came out challenging what the MSM was touting towards COVID were quickly buried.

What in the world was happening?

It became very clear to anybody who was watching closely that it was communism that was lurking under the surface throughout this entire process. It was communism that was sneaking in on the American people. And as such, those pushing communism did everything they could to begin silencing criticism. Throughout this process, it was almost impossible to say anything against the actions of Dr. Fauci, the WHO, or the CDC without being labeled as an irresponsible idiot.

Why was this done? Well, when it comes to a totalitarian state, as Hayek pointed out, "Everything which might cause doubt about the wisdom of the government or create discontent will be kept from the people."[3] He was talking about the growth of a collectivist state when he said this. With such, you have to keep the dissenters quiet – and by any means possible. Hayek had more to say on this. "Public criticism or even expressions of doubt must be suppressed because they tend to weaken public support." He would go on to add, "Every act of the government must become sacrosanct and exempt from criticism."[3]

This is indeed what we saw. Why else would there be a need to suppress *research*?

The scary thing about this though was that there were plenty of people throughout the USA who bought into everything that their TV was telling them. There were plenty of people who believed that the CDC, the WHO, and Dr. Fauci were truly working in their best interests. Hayek had something to say about these people as well: "The most effective way of making everybody serve the single system of ends toward which the social plan is directed is to make everybody believe in those ends. To make a totalitarian system function efficiently, it is not enough that everybody should be forced to work for the same ends. It is essential that the people should come to regard them as their own ends."[5]

Do you see that? For a totalitarian system to work properly, it must *convince* the people that what is going on is happening "for their own good". This is akin to the nations of the novel *1984* using bombs against their own people in order to convince the people that all of the war time measures that are in place are truly there for their own good.

Within Rand Paul's *The Case Against Socialism* he brings up the story of a family decimated by the Holocaust. I'll let Rand take it from here: "Jon asks the same question so many ask: 'Why didn't they resist more?' The answer, according to Jon, is that millions were condemned and executed for resistance, but the movement lacked momentum because the prison camps were very isolated and their horrific conditions kept secret."[6]

The irony behind Rand Paul's making such a point is that he would later disparage Americans who were actively doing so – by showing up to protests with rifles – even while communists were taking over the United States, even after Rand Paul was put into a hospital by a statist, even after Antifa had threatened him and his wife, even after America's freedoms were gradually being destroyed.

So what can ultimately be said about all this? Should criticism of the mainstream narrative be silenced? Should we use force to stop the mouths of those whom we disagree with? To better understand the answer to such a question we must delve into the philosophy of freedom.

To start, understand that "all silencing of discussion is an assumption of infallibility."[7] If you are to proclaim that somebody else can never say anything that is contradictory to what you believe, you are saying that you yourself – a human – are incapable of error. Perhaps prior chapters within this book will have proved to you by now the ridiculousness of holding such a position. If you're married, it did not take you long to realize that you weren't always right, did it?

The understanding that one has the capability of being incorrect is to possess a characteristic of humility. Those who are dogmatic in their approach and refuse to allow others to hold their own beliefs are succumbing to pride. It's interesting to note that it is often those with a "Tolerance" bumper sticker plastered on the butt of their vehicle who were the most intolerant when it came to "irregular" views on COVID.

Furthermore, as Mill pointed out, if we don't have freedom of speech, we don't have freedom of thought. It makes it a crime to even *think* a certain way. Do you like the idea of thoughtcrime being a thing? Do you like the idea of it being illegal to have an *idea* pop up into your head? To agree to such is to open the door for the criminalization of whoever disagrees with the government – perhaps indefinitely. To argue for the criminalization of thought is to say that you are a proponent of government brainwashing and "deprogramming" of political prisoners – what the great majority of prisoners under such a world would in fact be.

Do you like the idea of such?

How do we even get to this point? I would argue it is through effective propaganda. As FA Hayek pointed out, "If all the sources of current information are effectively under one single control, it is no longer a question of merely persuading the people of this or that. The skillful propagandist then has power to mold their minds in any direction he chooses, and even the most intelligent and independent people cannot entirely escape that influence if they are long isolated from all other sources of information."[5]

If you are a politician with an agenda, you can very easily get your goals met by silencing all criticism and then flooding the public with messages that help your cause. Given enough of such you'll even convince the educated – people who are by no means idiots – into supporting what you have to say! To summarize what Nazi minister of propaganda Joseph Goebbels said, if you repeat a lie often enough and loud enough, it eventually becomes a truth.

Once more, we can then return to what Hayek has to say. "It is not difficult to deprive the great majority of independent thought. But the minority who will retain an inclination to criticize must also be silenced."[8]

History has proven it's truly not hard to convince the greater part of a populace that a lie is truth. Consider the population of Germany in the 1930s. They were fully convinced that Jews truly were vermin – that they were spreaders of disease. That Jews polluted the genetics of a nation. And you are familiar with what this dehumanization of an entire race led to. Key to this process is the generation of fear.

The skillful propagandist must rely on fear to stir up the emotions of people. When emotions are stirred up – particularly fear – thought often goes right out the window. Beast-like actions follow. You could easily see this displayed in people throughout 2020. People were turned into sheep, willfully bleating whatever it was that their TVs told them to. Anytime there was some form of news or fact that violated what their TV told them (what they truly trusted, *not* the science), they could only reflect the actions of the sheep in Orwell's *Animal Farm*:

"Frightened though they were, some of the animals might possibly have protested, but at this moment the sheep set up their usual bleating of "Four legs good, two legs bad," which went on for several minutes and put an end to the discussion."⁹

This is why freedom of speech – freedom of thought – matters. The Founding Fathers understood that when you eliminate such, you set the stage for tyranny with a nightmarish level of power. They'd witnessed such from the Old World. They'd heard the stories about the Spanish Inquisition. They'd seen the thumbs screws, the iron maidens, and the rack. When freedom of speech is abolished, tyranny can do nothing *other* than grow. To argue against the freedom of speech is to argue for torture, random incarceration, government kidnapping, rape, genocide, and more. Those are all the eventual occurrences in governments without such *every single time.*

But What About Undeniable Truths?

The question can then be raised, "But what if we're talking about something that's indisputable? What if we're talking about the existence of gravity?" Freedom of speech can only help such a situation as well. Let's look at how:

Let's say we do have somebody arguing against irrefutable truth. Let's say we have somebody arguing that gravity doesn't exist. Should we silence even these people? For starters, consider that men such as Copernicus and Galileo were punished as heretics for arguing against what was once thought 'irrefutable truth'. Our knowledge of the world around us – of the universe – is constantly expanding. Where men once thought that it was impossible for mankind to fly, the airplane passes a shadow on. As priorly argued, humility permits others to speak. Only pride shuts others' up.

However, permitting people to voice opinions contrary to ours only serves to benefit ourselves as well. How can this be? By helping us to have a better understanding of our own position. Picture living in a world where nobody has ever attacked one of your beliefs. You will never have as thorough of an understanding of why it is that you believe what you believe. You would never be able to plug the holes, inconsistencies, and the like that you never would have noticed had not somebody else pointed them out to your attention.

At least in my own life, it was when I shared my faith with others – and they responded with sincere and curious questions that I'd never thought of – that I grew to have a better understanding of just what I believed, what Christ had done for me, and the like. You've undoubtedly experienced similar events whether we're talking about religion, politics, science, sports, relationships, or *any other subject under the sun.*

You must allow freedom of speech to flourish if you want there to be any evidence of a true search for truth. Otherwise, you honestly never know whether what you're being fed is food, or whether it's just a spoonful of chicken crap.

25

Why Capitalists are the Only Ones Who Care About Public Health

"If one wishes to uphold individual rights, one must realize that capitalism is the only system that can uphold and protect them." – Ayn Rand[1]
Those who want slavery should have the grace to name it by its proper name. – Ayn Rand[2]

I am fully convinced that it is *solely* those who are capitalists who care about the public health of a nation as a whole. No collectivist can show the same proof of care as any individualist can. It is simply impossible. While a collectivist most certainly may scoff at the idea that he doesn't care about others' health anywhere near as much as an individualist (aka, proponent of human freedom) does, the fact remains that it is so.

There are a number of reasons for this, and we will take a look at each one of them in turn.

Within socialism, communism, fascism, or any other form of collectivism the basic principle is to operate off of a system of theft. Collectivism is nothing more than a government approved system of looting a country – a morally reprehensible system.

Destruction of Incentive

It is a fundamental tenant of human nature that mankind acts out of his own self-interest. Adam Smith illustrated this point wonderfully in his groundbreaking treatise on the subject, *The Wealth of Nations*. Man doesn't spend years in training for a particular career, invest in equipment out of his own capital, wake up at 5:30AM every weekday, and put up with difficult customers for 8+ hours a day solely because he is feeling charitable.

He does such because he has his own personal goals he wants to accomplish. Goals such as funding his child's education, buying his wife a Valentine's gift, paying for his mortgage, investing extra money, saving for a new rifle, and so on. This is not greed. This is human nature. Man has the right to do with what he will with what he earns, and for another to think that he has any right over another man's wealth is to believe that one has the right to be a robber, and that the other has no right to be anything other than a victim.

One of the most egregious examples of this point can be seen throughout collectivist countries in the form of socialized medicine. When the government takes over the business of healthcare, the industry dies. Why would one want to spend 7+ years studying to be a doctor when you know that there are going to be incredibly long hours, lots of night shifts, difficult patients, the constant threat of being sued/jailed, the threat of catching a contagious disease, the threat of dying early due to the stress and difficulties of the position (doctors have a notoriously high rate of heart disease), and for minimal financial compensation?

You'd have to be a fool to sign up for such! Yet, that is literally the case when it comes to working in healthcare in a collectivist country. Roughly at the time of this writing, Venezuelan doctors make an average of $2.20/day, while Cuban doctors earn less than 1% of what American doctors make.[2]

If there is no incentive for the job in the first place – such as is the case with countries founded upon freedom, where a doctor rightfully can make six to seven figures per annum – then there will be nobody who decides to become a doctor. Even in countries that are based upon freedom, there is already a constant shortage of healthcare personnel such as nurses, nurse aids, surgeons, and physicians. When you take away the financial incentive that they receive to engage in such unattractive positions to begin with, you completely destroy a nation's ability to receive healthcare.

Malnutrition Runs Hand in Hand with Socialist Policy

Logic dictates that when a man realizes that he won't get to benefit from his work, he comes to the conclusion that it's better to not do any work at all (or as little as possible). As famed famer Joel Salatin says, "You may as well do nothing for nothing, if you're going to do something for nothing." History proves this concept even further. All we have to do is to look over the past 15 years to find a prime example. Let us examine Venezuela.

Maduro came to power in 2013 and quickly instated socialist policies throughout the country on a tremendous scale. And disaster of a tremendous scale quickly followed. Massive hyperinflation of necessity follows socialism around wherever it goes, with all that such implies. Part of this is food shortages and massive amounts of debt. This is exactly what we saw in Venezuela.[3]

Indeed, things got so bad there that the British newspaper Independent reported "the economic crisis in Venezuela is so severe that 75% of the country's population has lost an average of 19 pounds in weight..."4

Socialist policies bring hunger with them. Massive starvation is the norm for such nations, and once one fully realizes the full scope of negative health consequences of malnutrition (aside from death) it is hard to fathom how anyone could truly argue for the "beneficence" of a socialist-utopian state.

Lack of Medicine and Supplies

This goes hand in hand with a lack of healthcare personnel. Any form of collectivism whatsoever will quickly lead to a dangerous shortage of medical supplies within that nation. There are many reasons for this – the destruction of incentive, the theft of private property, hyperinflation, people clogging the system with non-urgent conditions that in other circumstances they would have taken care of themselves, government incompetence, increased need for health services as public health deteriorates, and so on – but the fact of the matter will be that there simply won't be the necessary equipment in order to keep people alive.

Look once more to Venezuela for proof of this fact. As Rand Paul points out in his *The Case Against Socialism*, "Hospital wards have become crucibles where the forces tearing Venezuela apart have converged. Gloves and soap have vanished from some hospitals. Often, cancer medicines are found only on the black market. There is so little electricity that the government works only two days a week to save what energy is left. At the University of the Andes Hospital in the mountain city of Merida, there was not enough water to wash blood from the operating table. Doctors preparing for surgery cleaned their hands with bottles of seltzer water. 'It is like something from the 19th century,' said Dr. Christian Pino, a surgeon at the hospital."[5]

Luis Avila of Venezuela sadly proclaimed, "My four-year-old daughter is dying of cancer, and there's no medicine here to treat her."[6] Other surgeons have stated similar conditions, saying that there are literally patients dying on the operating table not because they have untreatable medical conditions, but instead because surgeons do not have access to proper medicines and equipment.[7]

Brain Drain

As men realize that there is no reward for their effort, they naturally seek out areas where they will be rewarded. One of the natural consequences of such is brain drain. When engineers, nurses, doctors, inventors, scientists, and other highly skilled workers realize that they can make much more money, have much more autonomy, and have much more room for advancement within their field at a different location, they're likely to move there.

Thus, when you have a nation such as Argentina, the smartest, best, and most productive members of society are going to leave as quickly as they can. They'll go to other nations where there skills and abilities are appreciated and properly rewarded. The end result is the absence of men of merit from the original country: a brain drain.

Collectivist philosophies lead to such every single time. You cannot fight a law of human nature and expect to win in such a way. To argue for collectivist policies is to likewise champion the absence of surgeons, general practitioners, nurses, and others from current society (albeit unrecognizably). On the contrary, capitalism encourages those people to stay or immigrate.

If you want access to professional healthcare workers in your community, capitalism is the only way to ensure such is the case.

26

The Historical Proof of Capitalism's Success with Public Health

We've only to look back over the past few hundred years to illustrate the proof of such. It was throughout the twentieth century when the greater part of the world began to instate capitalist principles into their governments. Monarchies fell, aristocracies crumbled, as people realized the full benefits that could be brought about only via a republic.

It was during this time that childhood mortality plummeted from nearly a third of children dying before the age of five to less than 1% doing so in developed nations and 4.3% in undeveloped nations.[1] It was freedom that brought health, not statism, and all of the terrors that go with it.

It is when mankind is not plagued by constant theft, when he can truly reap the reward of all of his work, intuition, and creativity that an economy prospers and thus so does a nation's health. Once socialism of any form creeps in whatsoever, it is the beginning of the end.

Duty to Die

Collectivism is founded upon the principles of Marxism. There are those who are believers in what is called spiritual socialism, the idea that their religion justifies and perhaps even demands socialist behavior, but in the long scheme of things, these people are ultimately pawns for the paradoxically "true" Marxists. According to Marxism, the state reigns supreme, and the individual is nothing more than a means to an end. It is this understanding that has led to government-inspired genocide throughout the past 100+ years. Whether we are talking about the Holocaust, the Russian gulag system, Mao's Great Leap Forward, or about any other collectivist, the point remains that the genocide *was* logically consistent with Marxism, and thus has no right to be argued against by those who *thought* they were in favor of collectivist thought.

As FA Hayek pointed out in *The Road to Serfdom*, "Once you admit that the individual is merely a means to serve the ends of the higher entity called society or the nation, most of those features of totalitarian regimes which horrify us follow of necessity."[2] The reason for this is simple: you cannot put through collectivist policies unless you also "legalize" the force needed to enforce them. This is because there is a fundamental and intrinsic human understanding that theft is wrong. When an industry such as healthcare is nationalized, there are going to be those who resist. Doctors will operate on the black market, nurses will flee the country, and healthcare administrators will search for other jobs. None of this can be tolerated within a collectivist nation – healthcare workers are needed, and collectivism is in essence to argue that people do not belong to themselves, but instead belong to the state – and as a result a significant militarized police presence will be needed to stop all of these activities, and to stop them *hard*.

There can be no mistaking within a collectivist nation that such a behavior is acceptable, and therefore there need to be incredibly stiff penalties in order to keep others in their place. Again, FA Hayek illustrates this when he says, "...in order to achieve their end, collectivists must create power – power over men wielded by other men – of a magnitude never before known, and that their success will depend on the extent to which they achieve such power." (p165)

If you are going to rob people of their property, of their choice, and of their freedom, they are going to resist. Thus, you need an incredibly amount of power (aka, force) in order to force people to bend over and submit to your will. Aside from this exponential growth of military and police presence within the daily lives of the citizen, there will also be an exponential growth in the use of extreme measures in order to keep the public in line. This gets its source from two roots: collectivists must use extreme measures to ensure their programs succeed, and such occupations require that the worker be calloused.

Let's examine the aspect of the necessity of extreme measures within a collectivist society first. Collectivism is founded upon the idea that there is the ideal out there, and that mankind needs to reach it regardless of cost. This ideal is always a utopia. Historical determinism will often be used to argue that mankind is going to reach that utopia eventually, so why not do what we can to hurry along the process. If the utopian vision is that everybody has the right to a basic universal income, then we have to do everything we can to get that utopian vision to manifest itself. If that means nationalizing an entire populace's savings, capping earnings at $40,000 per year, and preventing citizens from moving overseas so that they can "do their part", then so be it.

There will undoubtedly be people who won't comply with this, but that quite simply cannot be tolerated. Those people will be viewed as coconspirators in the plot to derail the nation, and as such, they must be destroyed. FA Hayek points out once more, "There is always in the eyes of the collectivist a greater goal which these acts serve and which to him justifies them because the pursuit of the common end of society can know no limits in any rights or values of any individual."[3]

If our nation is in the quest to build Nietzsche's' "superman", and that necessitates the elimination of the "undesirables" from our society, then so be it. And thus, you end up with the Holocaust. Collectivism leads to the destruction of a man's humanity. He is no longer viewed as a human being with inherent worth and inherent rights, but instead as a resource to be used as the state desires. As such, it is only a matter of time within any collectivist society before it is discovered that those who cannot contribute to the state, or detracting from the state, and therefore must be eliminated. They have no inherent worth, and they are hampering "the greater good", which is the end all within collectivist thought.

And thus, you end up with people like a multiple sclerosis patient in Gothernburg, Sweden who was told that he couldn't receive a prescription for a new drug to treat his condition. Why? The new medicine was more expensive than the older medicine. Even when the patient appealed and said that he would like to pay for the medication himself, he was denied, because this would "set a bad precedent and lead to unequal access to medicine."[4]

In other words, "you do not have the right to live. You must suffer. That is the only fair option." But perhaps this is a little bit too abstract of an example for people to follow. If one cannot see how Sweden's example here is consistent with collectivist thought, then perhaps we can look at the murder of those with Down's syndrome, the elderly, the paralyzed, those with birth defects, those with learning disabilities, and others throughout Nazi Germany, Mao's China, and Stalin's Russia will perhaps paint the picture more vividly.

Let us now look at why only the calloused – those who delight in theft and murder – will end up being the ones who reign in a collectivist nation. Hayek once more has wonderful insight to shine on the matter. He first points out that collectivist nations require violence to reign of necessity. "...As there will be need for actions which are bad in themselves, and which all those still influenced by traditional morals will be reluctant to perform, the readiness to do bad things becomes a path to promotion and power."[3]

Hayek then goes on to point out what this requires. "...Of the duties of the authorities of a collectivist state that 'they would have to do these things whether they wanted to or not: and the probability of the people in power being individuals who would dislike the possession and exercise of power is on a level with the probability that an extremely tender-hearted person would get the job of whipping master in a slave plantation."[5]

To argue for a collectivist nation, is to argue to be placed under the thumb of sadists. Those who argue for such are no friend to either public health or mankind.

"Socialism means slavery."

The above title comes from a statement made by FA Hayek.[6] Socialism is nothing short of mankind's slavery to those who are within the realm of government. Moving on further, Max Eastman (a personal friend of Lenin) said that "Stalinism IS socialism." Within the same vein, FA Voigt, a

British writer had this to say, ""Marxism has led to Fascism and National Socialism, because, in all essentials, it is Fascism and National Socialism."[7]

So, if Stalinism and socialism are exactly the same - if fascism, naziism, and socialism are exactly the same – if they're not even two sides of the same coin, but simply the coin – how does the health of the nation fare with these systems put into place? How does a nation fare with a Josef Stalin, an Adolf Hitler, or a Bennito Mussolini at the helm? Considering that each of these men's names is directly tied in with massacre and holocaust, perhaps no other argument is necessary.

27

Eugenics

"If the state was going to plan the production of motor cars in the national interest, why should it not do the same for the production of babies?" – Jonathan Freedland[1]
"...no man or tribe may attempt to achieve the good of some at the price of the immolation of others." Ayn Rand[2]

Isn't it strange the steps people are willing to take in the name of public health? I want you to remember that question after you've made it through this chapter, and then ask yourself where else such happenings may apply.

If statism dictates that the state is the end all and be all – the improvement of which is the prime goal of all of humanity – then it logically follows that those who are a hindrance to such being accomplished need to be removed from the environment. While this may seem like a far out and extreme train of thought, keep in mind that such *is* at least logically consistent and that it *has* been reached by other men before.

Within a statist society, the only moral actions are those which benefit the state as a whole. Anything that helps to further such – regardless of how mortifying – must be viewed as an act of love and compassion.

Don't believe me when I say that others in the past have reached similar conclusions? Well, then let's take a ride through history together.

It was George Bernard Shaw (an incredibly popular socialist) who declared that "the only fundamental and possible socialism is the socialization of the selective breeding of Man." Here we have a man with considerable influence advocating for eugenics – the state's tinkering with its citizens' fertility and others' right to live. If you had a genetic defect that meant you were likely to have a child with a similar genetic defect (e.g. hereditary blindness), Shaw would argue that the state had the right to forcibly sterilize you so that you didn't bring such a blemish and burden (your child) to the light of society. That's not where it stopped, however. Shaw would also argue that you yourself should likely be eliminated from society. He didn't leave any questions of what this "elimination" would mean either, as he advocated later for the elimination of certain people by "lethal chamber".[2]

It seems as if Hitler and his Nazis followed Shaw's advice to the letter with *their* lethal chambers: the gas chamber.

But perhaps this is only an isolated example? Perhaps George Bernard Shaw acted alone in having such opinions? While the very presence of The Holocaust denies such a question from ever being made in the first place (for it was made by the National Socialist Society – what the acronym NAZI actually stands for), let's continue to examine the subject further.

Have you heard of William Beveridge? He was a very influential liberal thinker and advocate behind the concept of a welfare state. He argued that those with "general defects" – paralysis, blindness, learning disorders, colorblindness, etc. – should be denied the right to vote, freedom, and even the potential of fatherhood. To summarize, if you were born with or later developed some form of incapacitating injury, you should be forcibly sterilized, locked up in a cell, and then forbidden to have any say in the process of whether such an action was justified or not.[3]

The irony here is that those who are on welfare – often some of the strongest advocates for a welfare state – don't realize that this type of logic they support would eventually come back to haunt them in some truly terrifying ways.

What about Margaret Sanger of Planned Parenthood fame? Surely this icon of liberalism should be beyond reproach, no? One will hopefully change their mind when they read these words directly from her mouth, "The second step would be to take an inventory of the second group, such as illiterates, paupers, unemployables, criminals, prostitutes, dope-fiends; classify them in special departments under government medical protection and segregate them on farms and open spaces."

If you've ever read anything about what the US does when it segregates people groups onto reservations, you may not like what this ends up turning out to be. Once again however, there is a splash of irony throughout this argument. A socialist state breeds all of the individuals Sanger thinks need to be separated from the rest of society. Illiterates? Have you ever seen what public education results are like compared to private education? Compare the drop-out rates from both types of schools and you'll see what I mean.

Paupers? Socialist states, much like Venezuala, soon lead to starvation. Unemployables? Who else out there was deemed by the state to be an "unessential worker" after the *state* robbed them of their ability to work? Criminals? It's already been well-established elsewhere in this book that socialism only benefits those who are corrupt, ruthless, and willing to steal and harm. Prostitutes? If you look at the push for legalized prostitution that Kamala Harris is backing within the United States, I think you'll agree that such only encourages young girls to get involved in such a wicked profession. Dope-fiends? Europe – an entire continent of socialism – already has legalized drugs in many locations. Where drugs are legal, usage increases.

Sanger's ideas would have only *created* the very problem that she was wanting to eliminate all along. And what if you wanted to get off such a reservation, gulag, or prison? What if you decided that government treatment and services in such a location weren't what you wanted? According to Sanger, you would still be free to leave if you wanted to. But on one condition. You would be sterilized.[3]

Others have pushed similar theories. JBS Haldane, another prominent socialist and scientist, said, "Civilization stands in real danger from over-production of 'undermen'".[3] Such was an eerie echoing of German philosopher (Nietzsche) arguing about the destructiveness of the "undermen" within a society and how they hindered a state's inevitable and necessary growth towards utopia.

Beloved socialist economist John Maynard Keynes believed in eugenics as well, advocating for contraception for the working class in order to keep down their numbers. Why? Because they were too "drunken and ignorant" to quit producing children of their own accord, of course.[4] Once again, think about what such a statement implies. If a state is to mandate that a particular class of human needs to use contraception, how do you think they'll go about enforcing such? Will they blaisely hand out condoms and hope that people will use them? What happens when they find out that people resent such an intrusion into their private lives (no pun intended)? The same thing that will happen in every other case where the policy of the state cannot survive without brutality, of course. By resorting to forced sterilization in some manner or another.

And should it not cause some degree of hesitation in accepting the economic theories of a man who believed human freedom was of such little consequence or value that certain men and women could righteously be sterilized for the glory and good of the state? Who gets to decide who is that of little use or value? The answer will widely vary depending upon who you are asking.

I spent a bit of time in Asia in the past, and I can tell you without hesitation that all of Asia seems to hate each other. While in China, I foolishly went to play basketball in a dark alley with a bunch of strangers I'd never met before. Nobody from my group of tourists knew where I was. I couldn't read Mandarin, nor barely speak it. There I was, the sole white man in a sea of Chinese, in a dark, abandoned alley surrounded by young men. They asked me what I thought of Japan. I'm an avid World War 2 buff and answered that I wasn't a fan after what they'd done to Pearl Harbor.

The sole, choppy-English speaking guy there told me, "Good. If you say you like Japan, we beat you up."

My point is that if you ask the Japanese, they likely think the Chinese should be sterilized. Consider the Rape of Nanjing. Ask that question to a Korean, you'll get a different answer. Ask a Vietnamese, and they'll tell you another Asian nation.

So if forced sterilization is the policy, who gets to determine who gets chopped and who stays intact? The answer? Those in power. It is those who are able to cheat, steal, and murder their way to the top in a socialist country that get to decide who lives and who dies. It's as simple as that. And make no mistake, if you have the arbitrary power to decide who is of value and who is not, then you have the power to make eunuchs out of those whom you hate. It's all rather convenient really. That way they can't raise children with their heretical and seditious beliefs as well, right?

But let's look even further.

If to be an underman is a crime – one that is likely to be punished by death – then those who *create* such undermen will be guilty as well. The mother who gives birth to those whom the state deems disabled or undesirable, particularly the mother who does so more than once, is to be deemed as a threat to the utopia as well.

Another prominent socialist, Harold Laski championed this logic. "The time is surely coming...when society will look upon the production of a weakling as a crime against itself."[4]

If the end goal is the supreme power of the state, then to create a being that is flawed is to injure the state's end goal. It is to thrust upon the state a new responsibility where resources must be taken from some other project to now assist the life of "the weakling". In such a case, the weakling is likely to be forcibly destroyed (read: murdered), and if the mother and father continue to repeatedly produce such weaklings, the state will likely resort to the notion of forced sterilization on one or both of them so that such a "crime" is not continually committed against the state.

What Can We Glean?

Under no circumstances should a public health official ever advocate for eugenics of any form. It is a blatant violation of human rights and is outside the domain of authority of any human being on earth.

28

Little by Little

"It is seldom that liberty of any kind is lost all at once."
– David Hume

Freedom often dies the death of a thousand cuts. The ironic thing about this is that the knives are often held by those who claim to love freedom the most. As stated prior, public health is the perfect excuse to grow a state into a tyranny. This is especially the case when a populace is more than willing to jump on the bandwagon of slavery (often as a result of fear), slowly causing the death of capitalism, and therefore, freedom. As Thomas Pain stated in Common Sense, "...when republican virtue fails, slavery ensues."[1]

We must be on our guard to keep public health workers well within their sphere of duties. If we don't want to witness the death of freedom, we must not only hold public health workers, government employees, and politicians accountable for their decisions, but we must let them know when they have overstepped their rightful level of authority.

One of the chief ways that you'll see public health trample upon freedom is through the argument for an increased amount of safety. While we most certainly all want to know that we are safe, one never has the right to give safety to one man at the expense of another man. If you believe that rural folk are a safety risk to urbanites (due to country folks' individualism, patriotism, "privileges", etc.) you do not have the right to eliminate all farmers for the urbanites' safety. To do so places you in a similar situation as South Africa murdering and banishing white farmers simply because they possessed a different skin color than the rest of the population. All manner of atrocities can be argued for when safety is given as the necessary end goal. That has to be remembered, and it has to be remembered as well that no man has the right to infringe on the rights of another.

When these policies of government plunder – no matter how small – are put into place within a nation, time will quickly result in the populace developing into a nation of sheep. As FA Hayek pointed out, "...the policies which are now followed everywhere, which hand out the privilege of security, now to this group and now to that, are nevertheless rapidly creating conditions in which the striving for security tends to become stronger than the love of freedom."[2]

The argument for safety over freedom quickly becomes a character trait that is bred into the minds of those who would benefit from freedom most. The argument for safety will rapidly lead to a collectivist hive mind, where all manner of terrors will be brought about with the iron fist of governmental approval.

The early Americans faced a similar problem, and patriot Thomas Paine had this to say: "Ye that oppose independence now, ye know not what ye do; ye are opening a door to eternal tyranny."[3]

Every argument for safety is just a further opening of the door for tyranny to enter. Once you have decided that mandatory vaccinations are justifiable as a means of safety for the public good, you have now opened the door for an even further step where perhaps mandatory sterilization, mandatory euthanasia, or mandatory organ donation are necessary to further the end goal of safety.

Even the most innocent looking intrusions into the field of liberty for safety's sake can easily prove to be a nightmare in the very near future. This principle can be demonstrated by looking at Orwell's wonderful book *Animal Farm*. Within this book the farm animals have taken over the farm, and are turning it into a communist paradise. The pigs have decided that *they* are the leaders of the farm, and watch what happens after the dogs of the farm have had litters of puppies:

It happened that Jessie and Bluebell had both whelped soon after the hay harvest, giving birth between them to nine sturdy puppies. As soon as they were weaned, Napoleon took them away from their mothers, saying that he would make himself responsible for their education.[4]

Something innocent was brought about, but it quickly morphed into something else. Later within the story, a pack of vicious dogs appears out of nowhere quickly helping the pigs to cement their control over the farm.

At first no one had been able to imagine where these creatures came from, but the problem was soon solved: they were the puppies whom Napoleon had taken away from their mothers and reared privately. Though not yet full-grown, they were huge dogs, and as fierce-looking as wolves. They kept close to Napoleon. It was noticed that they wagged their tails to him in the same way as the other dogs had been used to do to Mr. Jones.[5]

An innocent intrusion into liberty can quickly grow to be a monster in the future. It doesn't matter if this intrusion is in the form of collectivist philosophy weaseling its way into the minds of millions, or of some other form of public health "need". One must always be careful of what they are introducing into either policy or legislation and to do their best to answer the question: "Does this decision intrude on the rights of another?"

For those who would believe that this is an argument against any type or form of law forever, I would refer you to John Stuart Mill's *On Liberty*. In this political essay Mill points out that there will be laws that will keep a man from doing anything he desires. A man may desire to dump all of his sewage into a nearby river, but in doing so he will endanger all of those who live downstream. Man does not have the freedom to live recklessly in such a manner, and when laws are created to prevent such from happening, they are not an intrusion within the bounds of freedom.

Man has a right to buy a car if he can afford it, but he does not have the right to drive that very car into another man's house. To do so is to damage the property and potentially the life of the man who lives within. However, Mills is not arguing for anarchy nor is he arguing for irresponsibility. Instead, he is arguing against government intrusion into spheres of human life that it has no right to meddle with in the first place.

It is not inherently wrong to have laws (passed through the proper channels) that keep men from dumping all of their sewage into a river. What is wrong is to issue arbitrary decrees that serve no purpose other than to serve as yet another tax or to intrude in spheres of human action where they do not belong.

Understanding this difference will permit the public health official to both protect the public health while simultaneously not causing nicks to human liberty as well.

29

Health Equality

"...people who accept collectivism by moral default; the people who seek protection from the necessity of taking a stand, by refusing to admit to themselves the nature of that which they are accepting; the people who support plans specifically designed to achieve serfdom, but hide behind the empty assertion that they are lovers of freedom, with no concrete meaning attached to the word; the people who believe that the content of ideas need not be examined, that principles need not be defined, and that facts can be eliminated by keeping one's eyes shut. They expect, when they find themselves in a world of bloody ruins and concretion camps, to escape moral responsibility by wailing: "But I didn't mean THIS!" – Ayn Rand[1]

It was shortly after the reign of fake American Obama that the term "health equality" (among other collectivist terminology) truly began to be thrust upon the American people. As Cleon Skousen pointed out in *The Naked Communist* and John Stormer pointed out in *None Dare Call It Treason*, America has long been infected with communists who have been stealthily injecting their ideology throughout America, gradually changing its laws, culture, philosophy, character, and ideals along the way.

However, it was during Obama's time that we began to see an acceleration. It was during those eight years that communism began to be injected into the US in much larger amounts. One of the ways that we saw this was through the argument for "health equality". This term is typically associated with the notion that America is an inherently racist nation. It is due to this systemic racism that there are health disparities throughout the US where a black man may not receive the same health outcome as a white man due to what we are led to believe is nothing other than the black man's skin color.

Questioning one's lifestyle, diet, smoking habits, monogamy, or other choices is never allowed to be brought up for analysis with the concept of health equality. In fact, to do so is frequently argued as being a *further* example of racism. The end result is the populace at large being coerced into the belief that if two different people of different skin colors end up with the exact same disease (e.g. diabetes), the non-white person will experience a worse health outcome than the white person simply because America is filled with racist white people. Nobody is allowed to question this conclusion without risk of ruining their reputation and (in some cases) outright acts of violence being perpetrated against their self or property in the process.

Understanding this, can it be argued that one can keep human rights in public health if they believe in the modern concept of health equality? If you believe that person A will receive a better health outcome than person B simply because of their skin color, what actions will you be led to perform? You will likely come to the conclusion that person A and all people like him must somehow be forced to support people like person B. You will likely come to the conclusion that that is the only moral way to proceed, and that as such, laws must be created (which will be enforced by men with guns, batons, handcuffs, and the ability to steal property and rob a man of his freedom) to forcibly *take* something from person A to give to person B.

Keep in mind that person A has in truth done nothing against person B. Person A simply takes care of himself better after receiving his initial diagnosis while Person B is adamant that they're going to continue living their life as they always have. Is it morally justified (because morality is *always* what we're talking about when we're discussing human rights) to engage in actions which rob Person A of something to give to Person B?

This doesn't necessarily have to be Person A's money (though that is typically always a culprit of theft as well). It could also include his opportunity. A single physician can only treat so many patients, and as such, many physicians only take on a set number of patients for their practice. Perhaps this doctor decides that health equality is a true issue in his community, and that he must do something to rectify the situation. As such, he decides that 50% of his patients will be of one skin color, 30% will be of another, and the final 20% will be of yet another heritage. Furthermore, this doctor decides that since white people are the most "privileged" within society, that they will comprise the final 20%. Giving any more of his patient population to white people would be to further the unequal access to healthcare, this doctor thinks.

It doesn't matter who calls the new practice to sign up with the doctor first. Once his quota for white people is reached, he's not willing to accept any more white people, and that is that. And all in the name of equality – in the name of justice.

Would such actions be right or would they be a violation of human rights? While the doctor most certainly has the right to run his business as he sees as fit, that doesn't mean his actions would be morally justified. Do people have any choice over what skin color and heritage they are, or are they simply born that way? If such is the case, to refuse service to people of one skin color is to refuse service to somebody simply because that is the way that they were born, is it not? Could this same doctor then decide that he no longer wants to treat anybody that is a red head (he'd had a bad experience with a red head in the past)? Could he not then also refuse service to somebody who was from a local college that he didn't like?

Those who work within healthcare should instead be focused on treating everybody the same regardless of who they are. If you are from New Jersey, you will receive the same level of quality care as somebody who is from Texas. If you are gothic, you will receive the same level of quality care as somebody who likes to wear yellow. If you are a man, you will receive the same level of quality care as somebody who is a woman. From my own experiences working within the field of healthcare and providing for patients, I don't see our system as having any problems with this. I never gave somebody a defective level of care simply because of their political beliefs, race, gender, nationality, religion, or anything else, and I never witnessed others do so either.

True, I most certainly may not like what those people believe in – I may even believe that they're wicked – but I will still give them the appropriate level of care. We've threatened people before with removal and banishment from our facilities before, but this was always due to those people either being violent, stalking staff, or being jerks - *never* due to any other reason. Provided you were willing to abide by a base level of kindness and respect for staff, you *would* receive your medical care. And even then, there were people who were hateful that we *still* were willing to care for. Being able to tolerate a certain amount of crap, and being able to discern when fear, pain, grief, or some other underlying cause was the origin of hatefulness comes with the job in the field of healthcare.

However, to argue that healthcare workers are inherently racist and won't give the same level of care to some simply because of their skin color is demeaning to all healthcare workers, and only spoken by the naïve or those seeking to cause strife and drive a political wedge with an underlying agenda into American society.

The problem with arguing for greater equality is that "all it tells us in effect is to take from the rich as much as we can."[2] Within the world of healthcare, all equality does is tell us to take from those we don't like as much as we can. Those who are viewed "rich" within the field of health – those who are deemed to be healthy – must be robbed of as much of their ability to receive service, of their access to a fair price, of an equal wait time for a procedure, and in other ways as possible in order that we may provide more of all these stolen items to those we believe are "poor" within the field of health.

While nobody is arguing against effective triage within an emergency room here – those who have a gunshot wound are going to need quicker access to healthcare than those who have sprained an ankle – that is not what is being argued for here. Medical triage and health equality are completely different, and to argue that they are the same is to not understand either. Triage is truly necessary to save as many lives as possible. Health equality is always a form of hate and robbery – it is always a form of systemic discrimination – against those who we believe have too much of something.

As such, you cannot keep human rights in public health while simultaneously arguing for health equality. You have the right to be treated as an equal, not the right to an equal outcome.

30

Are Sheddable Vaccines a Violation of Human Rights?

Do you have the right to refuse a medical treatment? Such is the very basis for this question.

Imagine you go to the doctor for a routine checkup, and the physician decides that you in fact are lactose intolerant. He then decides that you're going to be signed up for an experimental treatment for such with a host of potential side effects. You tell him 'no', you're not interested in such a treatment. You'll happily just avoid dairy.

But no, the doctor says you have no choice in the matter. You're being signed up for the experiment, whether you like it or not. You protest, to which the doctor grows combative. He presses a button on his pager and a group of large men in scrubs enter the room.

"We have a non-compliant patient, gentlemen," the doctor says as he points at you with his pen.

In an instant, the men with scrubs are upon you, pinning you to the table. You never noticed before, but there were straps on the table which they use to bind you to it. A nurse wheels in a small table with an array of instruments atop it – a syringe among them, you note.

As you scream and struggle against the straps, your arm is pinned firmly in place and a needle is jabbed into your arm.

You've just received the experimental treatment against your will.

What is your initial response to such a situation?

One of disgust, is it not? Perhaps fury?

You have this reaction because you have an inherent understanding that you have the right to your own body. It's your property, not others, and thus you have the right to make decisions that will impact it. After all, it's you that has to live with the consequences of decisions you make on your own body. If you have your leg amputated, it's you that has to learn how to maneuver with a prosthetic, deal with the pain, and shell out the money to stay upright, not the doctor, the nurses, or the politicians.

This is why informed consent papers exist. They came into being after the Holocaust when it was discovered the extent to which Nazi scientists and doctors experimented on Jews against their will. Twins were sewn together, men had perfectly fine limbs amputated, feet were sewn where hands were supposed to be, and so on. And all in the name of science. In the name of the 'public good.'

Understanding this, what should we think about sheddable vaccines? By that, I mean a vaccine that can be injected into one person but then hop to others who didn't want the vaccine as well. This is nothing new, by the way.

Eradicating Polio

As the world sought to eradicate polio from the planet, two scientists came up with a potential solution and roughly around the same time. One man created an injectable vaccine known as IPV. The other man created an orally administered vaccine known as OPV.

In developed nations, IPV was what was administered. It was a dead polio virus and permitted the injected to develop an immunity to polio. In undeveloped nations OPV was used. This version used a weakened, but live virus. One of the chief differences between the vaccines was that OPV could be shed. The thought process was that you physically can't get to every African village in the jungle. The infrastructure just doesn't exist.

If you can get just one member of that village to attend your OPV vaccination clinic though, they can then take that vaccine back to their village and shed it to everybody else there. Now the entire village is vaccinated against polio, and they don't even know it.

Examining the Ethics

But is such an idea morally justifiable? What you've just done in such a case is give a medical treatment to others without their consent. What if they didn't want the OPV vaccine? What if they had fears of Western medicine, not trusting your country? Do you still have the right to give them a medical treatment that they then don't want?

I would argue no.

It doesn't matter if you think it would be in the person's best interest. Why? It's not your choice. It's not your body. Just as you would take issue with a group of African villagers pinning you down so that the local witch doctor could shove cheetah excrement on your face (to cure you of your 'problem', of course), so they have the right to take issue with your sheddable vaccine.

Why Was Informed Consent Created?

By the subtitle I don't mean the justice of the idea of informed consent. That has always been. What I mean is the official recognition that informed consent needs to be a part of the way in which we perform any type of medicine whatsoever.

For those wondering, informed consent is the idea that a doctor needs your consent before he engages in any type of medical procedure on you. A surgeon can't just walk up behind you with a syringe, knock you out, and then proceed to do surgery on your liver without your ever knowing such was the plan.

You have to agree to the treatment or the procedure. Such comes from the inherent understanding that one's body is their own property. They are responsible for it, and as far as humanity is involved, an individual is sovereign over his own body. You do not have the right to make a medical decision for somebody else.

Just because you say, 'Cut that man open. Harvest his heart," does not make it so that a surgeon has the permission to do it on another human being. While, yes, the exception is made for the man brought unconscious to an emergency room, this is generally done because of what is considered implied consent. If a man has just suffered a gunshot wound to his abdomen, is bleeding out, and is unconscious, we can assume that he wants to live with little fear of being in the wrong. Surgery goes on for the man in order to keep him alive. The exception to this is with 'Do Not Resuscitate' orders or other forms of advanced directives.

While I agree there need to be safeguards put into place with this assumptive care ("Well we thought you would *want* the

COVID shot..."), overall, this is considered an acceptable practice.

The second half of informed consent is that the patient needs to have a thorough understanding of the procedure, risks involved, outcomes, and future consequences. Without telling the patient such, a physician is only doing half of his job.

But to get back to our original question, why was informed consent created as a modern concept? It came out of the terrors of the concentration camp. Post-World War 2, as Americans saw just what it was that Jews had been experiencing under captivity – sewing people together, injecting dye into peoples' eyes to change their eye color, forcing men to lay on blocks of ice to observe the signs and symptoms of hypothermia – a whole host of medical experimentations – that people realized this could not happen again.

The Nuremburg Trials began, Nazis were tried and executed, and the Nuremburg Code came into being in 1947. While I am against the greater part of international law, I don't think anybody will disagree that forced medical experimentation is a bad thing. If somebody wants to have their leg cut off and the situation warrants it, by all means, go ahead.

To cut somebody's leg off and to sew it to where their arm used to be – all as they scream in terror and writhe in opposition – is wrong. The Nuremburg Code assured that governments and doctors understood that they could no longer do such without facing grave consequences.

In reality, informed consent still remained nothing more than a concept. Tuskeegee, Alabama still inoculated men with syphilis – without their knowledge – and then monitored the men to see what would happen all the way to

1972. In many of these cases, the men's wives contracted the disease as well. Many of the victims literally rotted to pieces.[1]

In 1953, the CIA conducted MK-ULTRA, injecting people with LSD (against their will/knowledge) so that they could further study the effects of such. Throughout the 1950s the CIA pumped prisoners under interrogation full of 'truth serum' (scopolamine) to monitor what effect it would have as well.[2] The Soviet Union of the 1960s – 1970s regularly used pharmacological torture on its political prisoners. Insulin shock treatments, sulfazine, promazine, and haloperidol were all injected into prisoners under interrogation to cause fever, intense pain, extreme restlessness, and so on.

Many locations in the world are still conducting these same types of experiments and forms of torture on prisoners. Throughout the Middle East, and in China, where forced organ harvesting is a regular occurrence for political prisoners, this is the norm. One would be foolish to believe that Western nations are not performing similar actions on their own political prisoners at black sites around the globe. Under the scrutiny of the public eye, however, informed consent does seem to matter (in the greater majority of cases). Forced masking, forced shots, and forced PCR testing are all bringing this subject to the forefront of public discussion as the world at large recognizes what medical tyranny looks like and what it implies.

Is This All Theory?

Perhaps to the modern American this sounds as if it is a far-removed issue. It only occurred in Africa and the Middle East several decades ago, after all, right? So, who cares?

In reality, however, that is not the case at all. There is already much discussion within the scientific community as we speak regarding the use of sheddable vaccines in the future. This is touted as being a means to ensure that an entire community is vaccinated against whatever it is that we've deemed to be a threat without having to worry about the holdouts.

As of this writing, those who are "vaccine hesitant" are viewed as a strong problem within society. If you refuse to get the COVID shot, you are viewed as part of the reason that we can't "get back to normal". Never mind the fact that it is government action that is making it so that we can't get back to normal. We have to find somebody to blame, and so, those who refuse to get the COVID shot make good scapegoats. All future problems can easily be blamed on them. They can be used to justify future tyrannical actions.

However, what if you wanted to avoid all of that in the first place? Let's say that you were a staunch transhumanist and believed you had a moral duty to advance the evolution of the human race. You believed that gene modification was an excellent means of doing so. You realize that there's little to no chance that the public at large would ever consent to your plan, but that is due to the small-minded nature of the majority of the population. Few can see what the world could be as you do.

And as chance would have it, you've been successful in your funding of a gene therapy that can allegedly eliminate parasitical infections. *All* parasitical infections. The implications of such are huge, you believe. Giardia, malaria, tapeworms, pinworms – they will no longer be an issue for the human race. Mankind will have the ability to stay out at night, to inhabit swampy areas, to drink muddled water – and now, all without the risk of growing violently ill.

You haven't passed the process of the FDA as of yet, you only have 8 months' worth of research on the final product, but there's no time to waste! If you wait the full ten years to receive FDA approval, millions of people could die that didn't have to! You're not willing to let such happen, and were able to foresee that wasn't something you would tolerate either.

That's why you've made it so that your treatment is sheddable. By simply inoculating around 100 people or so, and sending them on planes throughout the continental US your calculations show that you can receive herd immunity against all parasites within ten months. The inoculation will shed, and shed, and shed with your end goal being reached.

Do you see how this could easily play out?

And researchers are already examining this as a possibility.

It's interesting to note that there are a wide number of allegations that the COVID shot already does the same thing – that it can be shed to others.[3] Thousands of anecdotal reports nationwide have crept in of women – even young girls – having very strange menstrual irregularities after being in contact with somebody who has recently received the COVID shot.

Whether such reports have any basis behind them or not is yet to be determined, but if true, this is a mass violation of informed consent. Nobody knows what the long-term effects of the COVID shot are. We do know that the spike protein spreads to every organ in the body, and that it particularly likes to nestle within one's ovaries. Could this result in future infertility? Mass miscarriages? Genital cancers?

Who knows? There's quite simply not been enough research.

But if the COVID shot is indeed a sheddable "vaccine", and if indeed this was known to be plausible beforehand, we now have a major criminal action that has taken place, that could potentially result in untold suffering (and death) for millions. And not only for millions currently alive, but potentially for future generations as well.

The Conclusion of the Matter

Perhaps now you see the point that I'm trying to make. For a wide variety of reasons – but ultimately due to an adult individual's right to make health decisions for their own body – should a sheddable vaccine be a concept that we would ever endorse as public health workers. To argue otherwise is to be a proponent of medical tyranny.

Afterword

"Is it just or reasonable, that most voices against the main end of government should enslave the less number that would be free? More just it is, doubtless, if it come to force, that a less number compel a greater to retain, which can be no wrong to them, their liberty, than that a greater number, for the pleasure of their baseness, compel a less most injuriously to be their fellow slaves. They who seek nothing but their own just liberty, have always the right to win it, whenever they have the power, be the voices never so numerous that oppose it." – John Milton[1]

It truly is hard to believe how far America has fallen within the span of only a year. Though the death of freedom in America has been a slow process since approximately the presidency of Woodrow Wilson, it increased exponentially under collectivist rule in 2020. David Hume famously said, "It is seldom that liberty of any kind is lost all at once." If he'd lived to see the coronavirus scam, he may have felt differently.

When it comes to crafting public health law (if one plays a role in such within their occupation), voting for public health law (the entire American public), or espousing various public health policies within one's conversations with friends, family, and colleagues, I cannot extol highly enough the importance of keeping human freedom at the forefront of the conversation. Do not compromise on stances where to do so violates decency. For as Ayn Rand pointed out, "In the field of morality, compromise is surrender to evil."[2] Perhaps no other philosopher has elaborated on the topic of compromise within politics to the extent that Ayn Rand has. She can also be credited with pointing out:

- "The rational (the good) has nothing to gain from the irrational (the evil), except a share of its failures and crimes."[3]
- "What is the moral status of an honest man who steals once in a while? ...What is the political status of a free country whose government violates the citizens' rights once in a while?"[3]
- "In any compromise between food and poison, it is only death that can win. In any compromise between good and evil, it is only evil that can profit."[4]

If you are willing to compromise on your morals, did you ever really have any morals in the first place? If you are going to argue for the theft and destruction of those who are lovers of freedom simply because you think that they are a hindrance to "the greater good", public health, and the utopian goal of a nation, then it is not the "hindrance" that is the problem and that will lead your nation to destruction. It is your own self.

For those who are having their freedom attacked under the guise of public health, I believe that we can glean some insight from those who came before us. First, understand that freedom is worth fighting for. Thomas Paine – the greatest writer throughout the American War for Independence – had a lot to say about this.

"Heaven knows how to put a proper price upon its goods; and it would be strange indeed, if so celestial an article as *freedom* should not be highly rated."[5] There will always be those who argue against human freedom, and I would argue that it is under slavery that mankind's miseries multiply. To fight for freedom is to prevent others from birthing increased suffering into an already fallen world.

Public health and freedom are not genres that a populace can idly step back from to live their lives as the wicked simply do whatever they want with them. "Those who expect to reap the blessings of freedom, must, like men, undergo the fatigues of supporting it."[6] If a man truly loves his children, would he not do what he can in order to prevent their having to suffer because he did nothing to stop the boulder that was coming to crush them? What can be said for the man who sits back and watches as his children are dragged into slavery? Can he trick himself into thinking that he is good?

Paine once more illustrated this: "If there must be trouble, let it be in my day that my child may have peace."[7]

To those that have reduced a nation to a state of slavery, I believe that they should be held accountable for their actions, as should those who would attempt to rob people of their human rights. "...If a thief break into my house, burn and destroy my property, and kill or threaten to kill me, or those that are in it, and to "bind me in all cases whatsoever," to his absolute will, am I to suffer it? What signifies it to me, whether he who does it, is a king or a common man; my countryman or not my countryman? Whether it is done by an individual villain, or an army of them? If we reason to the root of things we shall find no difference; neither can any just case be assigned why we should punish in the one case and pardon in the other."[8]

Aside from criminal charges being brought against those who have fought against human rights (much akin to the Nuremburg trials), I also believe that such agents should be barred from ever holding any form of public office within the United States ever again. If one has proved that they have zero understanding or care for human rights or for what it means to be an American, why should they be permitted to continue in their ability to make the lives who *do* know and care as miserable as possible? Why trust a child with a match if they've already burned down one house before?

Thomas Jefferson, in his Notes on the State of Virginia cautioned that the citizens of a nation guard against the growth of tyranny as well. "The time to guard against corruption and tyranny is before they shall have gotten hold of us. It is better to keep the wolf out of the fold than to trust to drawing his teeth and talons after he shall have entered."9 Is it not rather funny that the principle way public health works is via prevention, and the principle means that tyranny is fought is via prevention as well?

References

Chapter 1

1. Paul, Rand. *The Case Against Socialism*. HarperCollins Publishers. New York, NY. 2019. Pg. 170.
2. Rawles, James Wesley. *Patriots: A Novel of Survival in the Coming Collapse*. Ulysses Press. Berkeley, CA. 2013. Pg. 277.
3. Rand, Ayn. *Capitalism: The Unknown Ideal*. Signet Printing. New York, NY. 1967. Pg. 334.
4. *Ibid*. Pg. 326.
5. Rawles, James Wesley. Pg. 289.
6. Rand, Ayn. Pg. 332
7. Rand, Ayn. Pg. 334.
8. Hayek, FA. *The Road to Serfdom*. The University of Chicago Press. Routledge, London. 2007. Pg. 59.
9. *Ibid*. Pg. 112.

Chapter 2

1. KWQC TV 6 Web site. Bubonic plague warning issued in Lake Tahoe. Published September 5, 2020. https://www.kwqc.com/2020/09/05/bubonic-plague-warning-issued-in-lake-tahoe/
2. Wood, Patrick. ActivistPost.com. Amid COVID and riots, New York aggressively rolls out smart city tech. Published June 23, 2020. https://www.activistpost.com/2020/06/amid-covid-and-riots-new-york-aggressively-rolls-out-smart-city-tech.html
3. Frank, BN. ActivistPost.com. "Smart Pass" temp check/facial recognition promoted for businesses, schools, etc. What about privacy and safety? Published August 6, 2020. https://www.activistpost.com/2020/08/smart-pass-temp-check-facial-recognition-promoted-for-

businesses-schools-etc-what-about-privacy-and-safety.html

4. Maharrey, Michael. ActivistPost.com. Portland, Maine bans facial recognition technology. Published August 4, 2020. https://www.activistpost.com/2020/08/portland-maine-bans-facial-recognition-technology.html

5. Zernike, Kate. The New York Times. Christie faces scandal on traffic jam aides ordered. Published January 9, 2014. https://www.nytimes.com/2014/01/09/nyregion/christie-aide-tied-to-bridge-lane-closings.html

6. Frank, BN. ActivistPost.com. University partners with maker of "pandemic drones" to install COVID detection and social distancing systems. Published September 3, 2020. https://www.activistpost.com/2020/09/university-partners-with-maker-of-pandemic-drones-to-install-covid-detection-and-social-distancing-system.html

7. Weinstein, Mark. Huffington Post. What your Fitbit doesn't want you to know. Published December 21, 2015. https://www.huffpost.com/entry/what-your-fitbit-doesnt-w_b_8851664

8. Whitehead, John. ActivistPost.com. Virtual school dangers: the hazards of a police state education during COVID-19. Published September 15, 2020. https://www.activistpost.com/2020/09/virtual-school-dangers-the-hazards-of-a-police-state-education-during-covid-19.html

9. Yeboah, Kofi. ActivistPost.com. African Union turns to biosurveillance tech to curb COVID-19. Published September 14, 2020. https://www.activistpost.com/2020/09/african-union-turns-to-biosurveillance-tech-to-curb-covid-19.html

10. Wood, Patrick. ActivistPost.com. Privacy reset: UK readies digital ID cards for British citizens. Published September 4, 2020.

https://www.activistpost.com/2020/09/privacy-reset-uk-readies-digital-id-cards-for-british-citizens.html

11. Watson, Paul. ZeroHedge.com. Government advisers suggest giving COVID-free Brits "permission" wristbands. Published November 14, 2020. https://www.zerohedge.com/political/government-advisers-suggest-giving-covid-free-brits-permission-wristbands

12. This article has since been deleted. However, here was the original URL: https://www.zerohedge.com/medical/covid-19-vax-status-be-tracked-cdc-database-everyone-issued-vaccination-cards-according-dod

13. Tangermann, Victor. ScienceAlert.com. An invisible quantum dot 'tattoo' could be used to ID vaccinated kids. Published December 21, 2019. https://www.sciencealert.com/an-invisible-quantum-dot-tattoo-is-being-suggested-to-id-vaccinated-kids

14. Olson, Tyler. FOX 5 NY Website. Cities go to extremes with coronavirus quarantine crackdowns: Checkpoints, power shutoffs, steep fines. Published August 6, 2020. https://www.fox5ny.com/news/cities-go-to-extremes-with-coronavirus-quarantine-crackdowns-checkpoints-power-shutoffs-steep-fines

15. Wax, Gavin. ActivistPost.com. Media deems cashless society a "conspiracy theory" after admonishing cash use. Published August 5, 2020. https://www.activistpost.com/2020/08/media-deems-cashless-society-a-conspiracy-theory-after-admonishing-cash-use.html

16. Alderman, Liz. The New York Times. Our cash-free future is getting closer. Published July 6, 2020. https://www.nytimes.com/2020/07/06/business/cashless-transactions.html

17. Martinez, J. ActivistPost.com. Venezuela has gone cashless (and that's not all). Published August 14, 2020. https://www.activistpost.com/2020/08/venezuela-has-gone-cashless-and-thats-not-all.html

18. Paul, Ron. ZeroHedge.com. Ron Paul fears 'Fedcoin': a new scheme for tyranny and poverty. Published July 27, 2020. https://www.zerohedge.com/political/ron-paul-fears-fedcoin-new-scheme-tyranny-and-poverty
19. Durden, Tyler. ZeroHedge.com. Major Hollywood studio orders "AI-driven" face-mask detection robots. Published July 23, 2020. https://www.zerohedge.com/technology/major-hollywood-studio-orders-face-mask-detection-robots
20. GunBroker.com. PayPal/Venmo/Zelle/Apple Pay Policy on Firearms. Published December 24, 2021. https://support.gunbroker.com/hc/en-us/articles/224285428-PayPal-Venmo-Zelle-Policy-on-Firearms
21. https://americanmilitarynews.com/2020/03/ca-city-to-use-chinese-night-vision-drones-banned-by-us-army-to-enforce-coronavirus-lockdown/
22. Vibes, John. ActivistPost.com. Study finds some governments already using contact tracing apps for mass surveillance. Published June 20, 2020. https://www.activistpost.com/2020/06/study-finds-some-governments-already-using-contact-tracing-apps-for-mass-surveillance.html
23. Durden, Tyler. ActivistPost.com. Google says new "contact tracing" app to launch in coming weeks. Published August 1, 2020. https://www.activistpost.com/2020/08/google-says-new-contact-tracing-app-to-launch-in-coming-weeks.html
24. Broze, Derrick. ActivistPost.com. Newly released White House documents reveal effort to surveil Americans using contact tracing apps. Published August 7, 2020. https://www.activistpost.com/2020/08/newly-released-white-house-documents-reveal-efforts-to-surveil-americans-using-contact-tracing-apps.html
25. ActivistPost.com. Report: workplace coronavirus tracing apps institute dystopian mass surveillance by default. Published August 14, 2020.

https://www.activistpost.com/2020/08/report-workplace-coronavirus-tracing-apps-institute-dystopian-mass-surveillance-by-default.html

26. Frank, BN. ActivistPost.com. Studying sewage to track COVID?! No sh*t!. Published July 28, 2020. https://www.activistpost.com/2020/07/studying-sewage-to-track-covid-no-sht.html

27. Like many other articles, this one has since been deleted. Here is the original URL: https://www.zerohedge.com/technology/covid-19-and-pandemic-surveillance

28. Durden, Tyler. ZeroHedge.com. Michigan governor Whitmer goes full Orwell, demands full names, phone numbers for all restaurant customers. Published November 2, 2020. https://www.zerohedge.com/political/michigan-governor-whitmer-goes-full-orwell-demands-full-names-phone-numbers-all

29. Dumas, Breck. The Blaze. Vermont to question schoolchildren over Thanksgiving gatherings, and require quarantine for violators. Published November 24, 2020. https://www.theblaze.com/news/vermont-to-question-schoolchildren-over-thanksgiving-gatherings-require-quarantine-for-violators

30. OffGridSurvival.com. New York mayor Bill de Blasio announces snitch line to tell on social distance rule breakers. Published April 18, 2020. https://offgridsurvival.com/billdeblasiosnitchline/

31. Mass Private I blog. ZeroHedge.com. "Volunteer" Hawaiians turn "paradise on Earth" into an island of snitches. Published June 25, 2020. https://www.zerohedge.com/political/volunteer-hawaiians-turn-paradise-earth-island-snitches

32. Frank, BN. ActivistPost.com. Hotline to report people not wearing masks created for Ohio county residents. Published July 12, 2020. https://www.activistpost.com/2020/07/hotline-to-

report-people-not-wearing-masks-created-for-ohio-county-residents.html

33. Urbanski, Dave. The Blaze. 'Religious service,' 'indoor gun range' listed on Virginia health dept. 'online complaint' form to report COVID-19 'violations'. Published June 24, 2020. https://www.theblaze.com/news/religious-service-indoor-gun-range-complaint

34. Shilhavy, Brian. ActivistPost.com. Uber announces participating in contact tracing – they will turn you in to health authorities. Published July 20, 2020. https://www.activistpost.com/2020/07/uber-announces-participating-in-contact-tracing-they-will-turn-you-in-to-health-authorities.html

35. Watson, Steve. ZeroHedge.com. Backlash after UK policing minister encourages people to spy on neighbors for "COVID contraventions". Published September 16, 2020. https://www.zerohedge.com/political/backlash-after-uk-policing-minister-encourages-people-spy-neighbours-covid-contraventions

36. Field, Chris. The Blaze. Oregon's leftist governor tells residents to call police on neighbors who violate her new COVID lockdown edicts. Published November 23, 2020. https://www.theblaze.com/news/oregon-kate-brown-lockdown-rat-on-neighbors

Chapter 3

1. Yourish, Karen. The New York Times. One-third of all US coronavirus deaths are nursing home residents or workers. Updated May 11, 2020. https://www.nytimes.com/interactive/2020/05/09/us/coronavirus-cases-nursing-homes-us.html

2. Beer, Tommy. Forbes. CDC says possibly 'less than half' of positive antibody tests are correct. Updated July 26, 2020. https://www.forbes.com/sites/tommybeer/2020/05/2

6/cdc-says-possibly-less-than-half-of-positive-antibody-tests-are-correct/#cdf64772391b

3. Taylor, Sarah. The Blaze. CDC admits coronavirus may have infected whopping 10 times more Americans than previously thought. Published June 25, 2020. https://www.theblaze.com/news/cdc-admits-coronavirus-may-have-infected-whopping-10-times-more-americans-than-previously-thought

4. Sacca, Paul. The Blaze. Texas Department of Health removes over 3000 'probable' COVID-19 cases from overall count. July 16, 2020. https://www.theblaze.com/news/coronavirus-probable-cases-confirmed-texas

5. This post has since been deleted. It was originally at this link: https://nypost.com/2020/05/06/faulty-coronavirus-kits-suspected-as-goat-and-fruit-test-positive-in-tanzania/

6. Durden, Tyler. ZeroHedge.com. Tested 'positive' for COVID-19? Be sure to ask this question. Published December 6, 2020. https://www.zerohedge.com/medical/tested-positive-covid-19-be-sure-ask-question

7. Enloe, Chris. The Blaze. Shock report: Up to 90% of COVID positive Americans were possibly not even contagious. Published August 31, 2020. https://www.theblaze.com/news/shock-report-up-to-90-of-covid-positive-americans-were-possibly-never-even-contagious

8. Frank, BN. ActivistPost.com. COVID numbers inflated 600% due to false positives among university athletes: report. Published September 14, 2020. https://www.activistpost.com/2020/09/covid-numbers-inflated-600-due-to-false-positives-among-university-athletes-report.html

9. Taylor, Sarah. The Blaze. Texas county warns it will arrest COVID-19 positive people if they refuse to self-quarantine: 'You're going to be punished if you don't'. Published July 8, 2020.

https://www.theblaze.com/news/texas-county-arrest-covid-positive

10. Prestigiacomo, Amanda. The Daily Wire. 600,000 mistakenly told they've had covid: 'I have NOT been tested'. Published July 27, 2020. https://www.dailywire.com/news/600000-mistakenly-told-theyve-had-covid-i-have-not-been-tested

11. Yang, Ethan. ZeroHedge.com. New study exposes alleged accounting error regarding COVID deaths. Published November 27, 2020. https://www.zerohedge.com/medical/new-study-exposes-alleged-accounting-error-regarding-covid-deaths

12. Wolf, Leon. The Blaze. NYT: Fauci admits to deceiving the public about herd immunity because he wanted more people to get vaccinated. Published December 24, 2020. https://www.theblaze.com/news/ready-nyt-fauci-admits-to-deceiving-the-public-about-herd-immunity-because-he-wanted-more-people-to-get-vaccinated

13. Durden, Tyler. ZeroHedge.com. Gunshot to head, Parkinson's disease, deaths in Palm Beach incorrectly attributed to COVID-19. Published July 24, 2020. https://www.zerohedge.com/political/gunshot-head-parkinsons-disease-deaths-palm-beach-incorrectly-attributed-covid-19

14. Sacca, Paul. The Blaze. CDC: 6% of coronavirus deaths were solely from COVID-19. Published August 30, 2020. https://www.theblaze.com/news/covid-deaths-percent-coronavirus-cdc

15. Enloe, Chris. The Blaze. Woman has 'COVID-19 complications' listed on death certificate – but family says she never tested positive. Published August 15, 2020. https://www.theblaze.com/news/grandmother-death-certificate-covid-but-never-tested-positive

Chapter 4

1. Horowitz ,Daniel. The Blaze. Horowitz: if the panicmongers were consistent, we'd close the schools every flu season. Published July 16, 2020. https://www.theblaze.com/op-ed/horowitz-if-the-panicmongers-were-consistent-wed-close-the-schools-every-flu-season

2. Enloe, Chris. The Blaze. Groundbreaking study shows students rarely spread COVID, makes case for students returning to school. Published July 18, 2020. https://www.theblaze.com/news/groundbreaking-study-makes-case-for-students-returning-to-school-shows-kids-rarely-spread-covid

3. Horowitz, Daniel. The Blaze. Horowitz: NYT is 'surprised' by obvious lack of viral spread in schools that opened. Published October 20, 2020. https://www.theblaze.com/op-ed/horowitz-nyt-surprised-coronavirus-schoolchildren

4. Colen, Aaron. The Blaze. National teachers union authorizes its 1.7M members to strike if they don't like school reopen plans. Published July 29, 2020. https://www.theblaze.com/news/teachers-union-strike-reopen-plans

5. Colen, Aaron. The Blaze. NYC teachers won't show up unless every student and staff member gets a COVID-19 test, union threatens. Published August 19, 2020. https://www.theblaze.com/news/nyc-teachers-demand-tests-students-staff

6. Wolf, Leon. The Blaze. De Blasio tells New Yorkers: get ready for schools to close Monday, through the end of November. Published November 13, 2020. https://www.theblaze.com/hold-de-blasio-tells-new-yorkers-get-ready-for-schools-to-close-monday-through-the-end-of-november

7. Colen, Aaron. The Blaze. Parents say schools have reported them to child services for neglect if their kids miss online class. Published August 17, 2020.

https://www.theblaze.com/news/massachusetts-parents-say-schools-have-reported-them-to-child-services-for-neglect-if-their-kids-miss-online-class

8. Horowitz, Daniel. The Blaze. Horowitz: red state Alaska? Children will be forced to kneel for hours in school with masks and no recess. Published January 21, 2021. https://www.theblaze.com/op-ed/horowitz-red-state-alaska-children-will-be-forced-to-kneel-for-hours-in-school-with-masks-and-no-recess

Chapter 5

1. *Rawles, James Wesley. Patriots: A Novel of Survival in the Coming Collapse. Ulysses Press. Berkeley, CA. 2013. Pg. 379.*
2. Adams, Samuel. *The Rights of the Colonists as Men*
3. Smith, Adam. *The Wealth of Nations*. Coda Books. Arden, Warwickshire. 2012. Pg. 100.
4. The Wall Street Journal. FoxNews.com. Millions of Americans can't afford rent and eviction looms. Published July 17, 2020. https://www.foxnews.com/us/millions-of-americans-cant-afford-rent-and-eviction-looms
5. This post has since been taken down. Here was the original URL: https://www.activistpost.com/2020/07/yelp-over-50-of-restaurants-temporarily-closed-are-now-permanently-closed.html
6. Durden, Tyler. ZeroHedge.com. The number of permanent business-shutdowns is rising. Published July 24, 2020. https://www.zerohedge.com/personal-finance/number-permanent-business-shutdowns-rising
7. Durden, Tyler. ZeroHedge.com. "Financially devastated" – 83% of NYC restaurants unable to pay July rent. Published August 10, 2020. https://www.zerohedge.com/markets/financially-devastated-83-nyc-restaurants-unable-pay-july-rent

8. Durden, Tyler. ZeroHedge.com. Time to go all-in the "Big Short 3.0"? 80% of New York hotels on verge of default. Published November 13, 2020. https://www.zerohedge.com/economics/time-go-all-big-short-30-80-new-york-hotels-verge-collapse

9. Durden, Tyler. ZeroHedge.com. Sweden defeated the coronavirus without a lockdown – now its companies are reaping the benefits. Published July 29, 2020. https://www.zerohedge.com/geopolitical/sweden-defeated-coronavirus-without-lockdown-now-its-companies-are-reaping-benefits

10. Horowitz, Daniel. The Blaze. Horowitz: While Fauci tells US to 'hunker down,' Sweden's no-lockdown coronavirus results speak for themselves. Published September 15, 2020. https://www.theblaze.com/op-ed/horowitz-sweden-no-lockdown-coronavirus-results

11. Durden, Tyler. Activist Post. On verge of six-week shuttering, Australian small businesses beg: we can't survive another lockdown. Published August 5, 2020. https://www.activistpost.com/2020/08/on-verge-of-six-week-shuttering-australian-small-businesses-beg-we-cant-survive-another-lockdown.html

12. Rand, Ayn. *Capitalism: The Unknown Ideal.* Signet Printing. New York, NY. 1967. Pg. 322.

13. *Ibid.* Pg. 203.

14. Hayek, FA. *The Road to Serfdom.* The University of Chicago Press. Routledge, London. 2007. Pg. 124.

15. *Ibid.* Pg. 147.

16. *Ibid.* Pg. 130.

17. *Ibid.* Pg. 138.

18. Smith, Adam. *The Wealth of Nations.* Coda Books. Arden, Warwickshire. 2012. Pg. 134.

19. Paine, Thomas. *The Constitution of the United States of America and Selected Writings of the Founding Fathers: Common Sense.* Barnes and Noble. New York, NY. 2012. Pg. 146.

20. Smith, Adam. *The Wealth of Nations.* Coda Books. Arden, Warwickshire. 2012. Pg. 113.

21. Hayek, FA. *The Road to Serfdom*. Page. 158.
22. Watson, Paul Joseph. ZeroHedge.com. Infectious diseases expert says UK lockdown is not working. Published January 22, 2021. https://www.zerohedge.com/covid-19/infectious-diseases-expert-says-uk-lockdown-not-working
23. Rand, Ayn. *Capitalism: The Unknown Ideal*. Pg. 336.

Chapter 6

1. Bastiat, Frederic. *The Law*. Tribeca Books. Auburn, AL. 2007. Pg. 19.
2. Mill, John Stuart. *On Liberty*. AHM Publishing Corporation. Arlington Heights, IL. 1947. Pg. 10.
3. Payzer, Genevieve. Coursework submitted to Stanford University. Nazi sterilization experiments. Published March 27, 2017. http://large.stanford.edu/courses/2017/ph241/payzer2/
4. Tate, Aden. *The Faithful Prepper: A Christian's Perspective on Prepping*. Prepper Press. 2019. Page 168.
5. Snyder, Michael. ZeroHedge.com. Can employers fire any employees that choose not to take the COVID vaccine? Published December 4, 2020. https://www.zerohedge.com/medical/can-employers-fire-any-employees-choose-not-take-covid-vaccine
6. Durden, Tyler. TheBurningPlatform.com. Red flags soar as Big Pharma will be exempt from COVID-19 vaccine liability claims. Published August 1, 2020. https://www.theburningplatform.com/2020/08/01/red-flags-soar-as-big-pharma-will-be-exempt-from-covid-19-vaccine-liability-claims/
7. Peeples, Lynne. Proceedings of the National Academy of Sciences of the United States of America. News feature: avoiding pitfalls in the pursuit of a COVID-19 vaccine. Published April 14, 2020. https://www.pnas.org/content/117/15/8218

8. Durden, Tyler. ZeroHedge.com. Australia cancels COVID vaccine trial over 'unexpected' false positives for HIV. Published December 11, 2020. https://www.zerohedge.com/medical/australia-cancels-covid-vaccine-trial-over-unexpected-false-positives-hiv

9. Durden, Tyler. ZeroHedge.com. FDA says 2 participants in Pfizer COVID vaccine trial have died. Published December 8, 2020. https://www.zerohedge.com/geopolitical/fda-says-2-participants-pfizer-covid-vaccine-trial-have-died

10. Durden, Tyler. ZeroHedge.com. AstraZeneca shares plunge as COVID vaccine study put on hold due to "adverse reaction". Published September 8, 2020. https://www.zerohedge.com/medical/astrazeneca-shares-plunge-covid-vaccine-study-put-hold-due-adverse-reaction

11. Armstrong, Martin. TheBurningPlatform.com. COVID-19 vaccine warnings women should not get pregnant for at least 2 months after vaccination. Publisehd December 9, 2020. https://www.theburningplatform.com/2020/12/09/covid-19-vaccine-warnings-women-should-not-get-pregnant-for-at-least-2-months-after-vaccination/

12. CFT Team. ChristiansForTruth.com. Researchers advise men to freeze sperm prior to receiving COVID vaccine over concerns it may lead to sterility. Published December 25, 2020. https://christiansfortruth.com/researchers-advise-men-to-freeze-sperm-prior-to-receiving-covid-vaccine-over-concerns-it-may-cause-sterility/

13. Taylor, Sarah. The Blaze. UK issues allergy alert over COVID vaccine after 2 fall ill, now says vaccine should only be given where resuscitation measures are available. Published December 9, 2020. https://www.theblaze.com/news/uk-allergy-alert-covid-vaccine

14. To find video evidence of such statements, visit my Telegram page at Aden Tate. There I have catalogued a wide variety of ills due to the COVID shot.

15. TVR Staff. TheVaccineReaction.org. Only one percent of vaccine reactions reported to VAERS. Published January 9, 2020. https://thevaccinereaction.org/2020/01/only-one-percent-of-vaccine-reactions-reported-to-vaers/

16. The Washington Standard. Operation Warp Speed general: "Upon emergency use authorization, all of America must receive vaccine within 24 hours" (video). Published November 19, 2020. https://thewashingtonstandard.com/operation-warp-speed-general-upon-emergency-use-authorization-all-of-america-must-receive-vaccine-within-24-hours-video/

17. Sun, Deedee. KIRO 7 News. FBI warns of harsh penalty that comes with faking COVID vaccination cards. Published May 7, 2021. https://www.kiro7.com/news/local/fbi-warns-harsh-penalty-that-comes-with-faking-covid-vaccination-cards/SGBUBY5OK5GKZMIWU5QDBPEV2A/

18. Schachtel, Jordan. American Institute for Economic Research. Papers, Please! Oregon now requires 'proof of vaccination.' Published May 25, 2021. https://www.aier.org/article/papers-please-oregon-now-requires-proof-of-vaccination/

19. Durden, Tyler. ZeroHedge.com. UK's Boris Johnson says won't make COVID vaccination compulsory. Published November 23, 2020. https://www.zerohedge.com/geopolitical/boris-johnson-says-wont-make-covid-vaccination-compulsory

20. Durden, Tyler. ZeroHedge.com. British elite army unit to spy on and combat 'anti-vax militants': Sunday Times. Published December 1, 2020. https://www.zerohedge.com/political/british-elite-army-unit-spy-combat-anti-vaxxers-sunday-times

21. Watson, Paul. ZeroHedge.com. Chief medical officer says Canadians who refuse vaccine won't have "freedom to move around". Published December 5, 2020. https://www.zerohedge.com/political/chief-medical-officer-says-canadians-who-refuse-vaccine-wont-have-freedom-move-around
22. Mill, John Stuart. *On Liberty*. AHM Publishing Corporation. Arlington Heights, IL. 1947. Pg. 4-5
23. Taylor, Sarah. The Blaze. Qantas airlines says if you don't have a COVID vaccination, you probably won't be able to fly. Published November 24, 2020. https://www.theblaze.com/news/qantas-airlines-require-covid-vaccination
24. Watson, Steve. ZeroHedge.com. NJ lawmaker wants mandatory COVID shot for all kids without exemption. Published December 11, 2020. https://www.zerohedge.com/political/nj-lawmaker-wants-mandatory-covid-shot-all-kids-without-exemption
25. Stave, Mat. LifeNews.com. Colorado bill would require "re-education" classes for parents who refuse coronavirus vaccine. Published June 9, 2020. https://www.lifenews.com/2020/06/09/colorado-bill-would-require-re-education-classes-for-parents-who-refuse-coronavirus-vaccine/#.Xun8DI4eLpo.twitter
26. Colen, Aaron. The Blaze. COVID-19 antibodies fade quickly after infection, prompting questions about long-term immunity, study finds. Published June 22, 2020. https://www.theblaze.com/news/covid-19-antibodies-fade-quickly-prompting-questions-about-long-term-immunity-study
27. Taylor, Sarah. The Blaze. New study on COVID-19 antibodies suggests that immunity fades within weeks, authors say it puts a 'nail in the coffin' of herd immunity. Published July 13, 2020. https://www.theblaze.com/news/new-study-dashes-concept-of-herd-immunity-in-covid-19-patients

28. Durden, Tyler. ZeroHedge.com. 'It will never be licensed in the US' – Analyst warns AstraZeneca vaccine efficacy "embellished". Published November 23, 2020. https://www.zerohedge.com/geopolitical/it-will-never-be-licensed-us-analyst-warns-astrazeneca-vaccine-efficacy-embellished

Chapter 7

1. Martino, Joe. ZeroHedge.com. US government and Yale hold trials on how best to "persuade" Americans to take COVID-19 vaccine. Published August 5, 2020. https://www.zerohedge.com/political/us-govt-yale-hold-trials-how-best-persuade-americans-take-covid-19-vaccine
2. Urbanski, Dave. The Blaze. 'Board of shame' could come for businesses that ignore COVID-19 mask rule, Democratic mayor says. Published June 25, 2020. https://www.theblaze.com/news/board-of-shame-could-come-for-businesses-that-ignore-covid-19-mask-rule-democratic-mayor-says
3. Durden, Tyler. ZeroHedge.com. West Virginia offers gun, trucks, and piles of cash to encourage vaccinations. Published June 2, 2021. https://www.zerohedge.com/political/west-virginia-offers-gun-and-truck-prizes-vaccinated-residents
4. Durden, Tyler. ZeroHedge.com. Ohio offers weekly million dollar lottery prize for vaccinated people. Published May 13, 2021. https://www.zerohedge.com/covid-19/ohio-offers-weekly-million-dollar-lottery-prize-vaccinated-people

Chapter 8

1. Rand, Ayn. *Capitalism: The Unknown Ideal.* Signet Printing. New York, NY. 1967. Pg. 330.

2. Kiriakou, John. Institute for Policy Studies. Three Felonies a Day. Published June 10, 2015. https://ips-dc.org/three-felonies-day/

3. Fry, Hannah. The LA Times. Paddle boarder chased by boat, arrested in Malibu after flouting coronavirus closures. Published April 3, 2020. https://www.latimes.com/california/story/2020-04-03/paddle-boarder-arrested-in-malibu-after-flouting-coronavirus-closures

4. Urbanski, Dave. The Blaze. Not wearing a mask in public is 'act of domestic terrorism,' LA County health officer declares. Published December 1, 2020. https://www.theblaze.com/news/not-wearing-mask-in-public-is-act-of-domestic-terrorism-la-county-health-officer-declares

5. Vibes, John. ActivistPost.com. Colorado town threatens up to a year in jail for people who don't wear masks. Published July 10, 2020. https://www.activistpost.com/2020/07/colorado-town-threatens-up-to-a-year-in-jail-for-people-who-dont-wear-masks.html

6. SovereignMan.com. Leaving tire marks on the road is now a hate crime. Published July 17, 2020. https://www.sovereignman.com/trends/leaving-tire-marks-on-the-road-is-now-a-hate-crime-28260/

7. Enloe, Chris. The Blaze. Nashville councilwoman wants attempted murder charges for people who don't wear face mask, pass on COVID-19. Published August 8, 2020. https://www.theblaze.com/news/nashville-councilwoman-wants-attempted-murder-charges-for-people-who-dont-wear-mask-pass-on-covid-19

8. Olson, Tyler. Fox 5 NY. Cities go to extremes with coronavirus quarantines, crackdowns: Checkpoints, power shutoffs, steep fines. Published August 6, 2020. https://www.fox5ny.com/news/cities-go-to-extremes-with-coronavirus-quarantine-crackdowns-checkpoints-power-shutoffs-steep-fines

9. Colen, Aaron. The Blaze. Police haul man out of school board meeting about mask mandates for not wearing a mask. Published September 15, 2020. https://www.theblaze.com/news/police-school-board-meeting-maskless-man
10. Field, Chris. The Blaze. North Korea publicly executes citizen who violated COVID-19 quarantine edicts: report. Published December 4, 2020. https://www.theblaze.com/news/north-korea-publicly-executes-citizen-who-violated-covid-quarantine
11. Carroll, Patrick. ActivistPost.com. Canadian restaurant owner charged with "trespassing" after reopening in defiance of lockdown orders. Published December 9, 2020. https://www.activistpost.com/2020/12/canadian-restaurant-owner-charged-with-trespassing-after-reopening-in-defiance-of-lockdown-orders.html
12. Paul, Rand. *The Case Against Socialism*. HarperCollins Publishers. New York, NY. 2019. Pg. 138.
13. Durden, Tyler. ZeroHedge.com. People who reject face masks more likely to be sociopaths: study. Published September 2, 2020. https://www.zerohedge.com/political/people-who-reject-face-masks-more-likely-be-sociopaths-study
14. Sacca, Paul. The Blaze. Couple arrested and removed from NYC ferry in handcuffs for not wearing face masks: 'We're being targeted'. Published September 6, 2020. https://www.theblaze.com/news/couple-arrested-not-wearing-mask-nyc-ferry
15. Bovard, James. ZeroHedge.com. Deceit and demagoguery in Montgomery County, Maryland. Published August 8, 2020. https://www.zerohedge.com/political/deceit-and-demagoguery-montgomery-county-maryland
16. Pandolfo, Chris. The Blaze. NJ gym owner has been fined over 1.2 million for defying lockdown. No COVID-19 cases have been traced to his gym. Published

December 10, 2020. https://www.theblaze.com/news/nj-gym-owner-fined-defying-lockdown

17. Durden, Tyler. ZeroHedge.com. NJ gym owners accuse gov of "flexing his little tyrant muscles" after being arrested for contempt. Published July 27, 2020. https://www.zerohedge.com/political/new-jersey-gym-owners-arrested-defying-court-order-close

18. Enloe, Chris. The Blaze. New Jersey gym owners, who were arrested for defying shutdown, kick down gov't-installed barriers to reopen. Published August 1, 2020. https://www.theblaze.com/news/new-jersey-gym-owners-who-were-arrested-for-defying-shutdown-kick-down-govt-installed-barriers-to-reopen

19. Shiver, Phil. The Blaze. Colorado study finds no link between gyms and coronavirus outbreaks. Published December 23, 2020. https://www.theblaze.com/news/colorado-study-gyms-coronavirus

20. Taylor, Sarah. The Blaze. UK police will enter private homes and break up Christmas gatherings if they violate lockdown rules. Published October 28, 2020. https://www.theblaze.com/news/police-private-homes-christmas-gatherings

21. Bastiat, Frederic. *The Law*. Tribeca Books. Auburn, AL. 2007. Pg. 8.

22. Skousen, Paul. *The Naked Socialist*. The Ensign Publishing Company. Riverton, UT. 2014. Pg. 146.

23. Duffy, Peter. *The Bielski Brothers*. Harper Perennial. 2004. Pg. 124.

Chapter 9

1. Adams, Samuel. *American Independence*.

2. Dumas, Breck. The Blaze. Pelosi insists it isn't her fault she violated coronavirus restrictions, actually says 'I think that this salon owes me an apology'. Published September 2, 2020.

https://www.theblaze.com/news/pelosi-blames-salon-she-was-caught-in-during-shutdown-says-they-owe-her-an-apology

3. This post seems to have been deleted. It used to be available at: https://www.theburningplatform.com/2020/09/01/pelosi-used-shuttered-san-francisco-hair-salon-for-blow-out-owner-calls-it-slap-in-the-face/

4. The Spectator. Published May 4, 2020. DOJ sides with church suing Virginia governor Northam after pastor threatened with fine, jail time for holding 16-person service. https://thespectator.info/2020/05/04/doj-sides-with-church-suing-virginia-governor-northam-after-pastor-threatened-with-fine-jail-time-for-holding-16-person-service/

5. Urbanski, Dave. The Blaze. 'Religious service,' 'indoor gun range' listed on Virginia health dept. 'online complaint' form to report COVID-19 'violations. Published June 24, 2020. https://www.theblaze.com/news/religious-service-indoor-gun-range-complaint

6. Feuerherd, Ben. The New York Post. Pennsylvania health official moved mother from nursing home as deaths skyrocketed. Published May 13, 2020. https://nypost.com/2020/05/13/pennsylvania-health-official-moved-mother-from-nursing-home/

7. Washington DC government. Mayor's Order 2020-080: wearing of masks in the District of Columbia to prevent spread of COVID-19. Published July 22, 2020. https://coronavirus.dc.gov/maskorder

8. Durden, Tyler. ZeroHedge.com. "I have a right to make sure that my home is secure": Chicago mayor Lightfoot defends ban on protestors on her block. Published August 21, 2020. https://www.zerohedge.com/markets/i-have-right-make-sure-my-home-secure-chicago-mayor-lightfoot-defends-ban-protesters-her

9. Shiver, Phil. The Blaze. Report: with Chicago police already stretched thin, Mayor Lightfoot stations over 100 cops outside home, bans protests on her block to protect herself. Published August 20, 2020. https://www.theblaze.com/news/protests-banned-police-guard-chicago-mayors-home

10. Garcia, Carlos. The Blaze. Democratic Chicago official caught violating lockdown rules at his restaurant, calls it an 'error' in judgment. Published December 7, 2020. https://www.theblaze.com/news/chicago-tunney-lockdown-coronavirus-hypocrisy

11. Durden, Tyler. ZeroHedge.com. Minneapolis City Council members enjoy costly private security detail as push to "defund the police" continues. Published June 27, 2020. https://www.zerohedge.com/political/minneapolis-city-council-members-enjoy-costly-private-security-detail-push-defund-police

12. Durden, Tyler. ZeroHedge.com. "I humbly ask for your forgiveness" – yet another Democrat leader busted breaking his own COVID rules. Published November 26, 2020. https://www.zerohedge.com/political/i-humbly-ask-your-forgiveness-yet-another-democrat-leader-busted-breaking-his-own-covid

13. Durden, Tyler. ZeroHedge.com. Philadelphia mayor shamed after eating indoors in Maryland while his city remains shut down. Published September 1, 2020. https://www.zerohedge.com/markets/philadelphia-mayor-shamed-after-eating-indoors-maryland-while-his-city-remains-shut-down

14. Husebo, Wendell. Breitbart. Anniversary: Anthony Fauci appeared maskless at Nationals baseball game, contradicting own advice. Published July 23, 2021. https://www.breitbart.com/politics/2021/07/23/anniversary-anthony-fauci-appeared-maskless-nationals-baseball-game-contradicting-own-advice/

15. Watson, Paul. ZeroHedge.com. Doctor who demanded mandatory mask law pictured partying maskless on boat

surrounded by bikini-clad women. Published November 26, 2020. https://www.zerohedge.com/political/doctor-who-demanded-mandatory-mask-law-pictured-partying-maskless-boat-surrounded-bikini

16. Durden, Tyler. ZeroHedge.com. "Lockdowns for thee, but not for me" – Newsom, Pelosi attend dinner parties while US COVID cases explode. Published November 14, 2020. https://www.zerohedge.com/political/lockdowns-thee-not-me-gavin-pelosi-attend-dinner-parties-while-us-covid-cases-explode

17. Dumas, Breck. The Blaze. Gavin Newsom responds after getting busted attending large dinner party against his own advice. Published November 13, 2020. https://www.theblaze.com/news/gavin-newsom-responds-after-getting-busted-attending-large-dinner-party-against-his-own-advice

18. Enloe, Chris. The Blaze. San Francisco's Dem mayor says more severe COVID-19 restrictions on the way after being caught dining at fancy restaurant. Published December 2, 2020. https://www.theblaze.com/news/san-francisco-mayor-more-severe-covid-restrictions

19. Garcia, Carlos. The Blaze. San Francisco mayor attended birthday party at the same exclusive restaurant where Gavin Newsom was caught dining maskless. Published December 1, 2020. https://www.theblaze.com/news/london-breed-dining-hypocrisy-lockdown

20. Widburg, Andrea. AmericanThinker.com. Another Democrat is caught violating the rules she imposes on others. Published December 1, 2020. https://www.americanthinker.com/blog/2020/12/another_democrat_is_caught_violating_the_rules_she_imposes_on_others.html https://www.theblaze.com/news/la-county-official-votes-to-ban-outdoor-dines-outdoors

21. Shiver, Phil. The Blaze. San Jose mayor joins elderly parents and 'unknown number' of others for Thanksgiving after telling residents to 'cancel' gatherings. Published December 1, 2020. https://www.theblaze.com/news/san-jose-mayor-thanksgiving-covid-hypocrisy

22. Pandolfo, Chris. The Blaze. San Jose mayor apologizes for breaking COVID rules after telling others to follow them. Published December 1, 2020. https://www.theblaze.com/news/san-jose-mayor-apologizes-for-breaking-covid-rules

23. Hogan, Bernadette. The New York Post. Gov. Cuomo floats hosting his elderly mom for Thanksgiving, sparks uproar. Published November 23, 2020. https://nypost.com/2020/11/23/cuomo-floats-hosting-his-mom-for-thanksgiving-setting-off-an-uproar/

24. Durden, Tyler. Democratic Austin mayor urged citizens "not to relax...stay home" while vacationing in Cabo. Published December 2, 2020. https://www.zerohedge.com/political/austin-mayor-urged-citizens-not-relax-stay-home-while-vacationing-cabo

25. Dumas, Breck. The Blaze. Jen Psaki justifies Biden violating his own mask mandate by saying the president was 'celebrating'. Published January 21, 2021. https://www.theblaze.com/news/jen-psaki-justifies-biden-violating-his-own-mask-mandate-saying-president-was-celebrating

26. Enloe, Chris. The Blaze. Restaurant owner reduced to tears over Dem hypocrisy: her business is shut down, but Hollywood gets pass. Published December 5, 2020. https://www.theblaze.com/news/restaurant-owner-reduced-to-tears-blasts-dem-leaders-for-shutting-her-restaurant-giving-hollywood-pass

27. Durden, Tyler. ZeroHedge.com. Owner of NYC bar arrested days after declaring "autonomous zone" to dodge pandemic restrictions. Published December 3,

2020. https://www.zerohedge.com/medical/owner-nyc-bar-arrested-days-after-declaring-autonomous-zone-dodge-pandemic-restrictions
28. Adams, Samuel. *The Rights of the Colonists as Men.*
29. Paine, Thomas. *Common Sense.*

Chapter 10

1. Ebbs, Stephanie. FDA revokes permission to treat COVID-19 with hydroxychloroquinine, drug previously touted by Trump. Published June 15, 2020. https://abcnews.go.com/Politics/fda-revokes-permission-treat-covid-19-hydroxychloroquine-drug/story?id=71259078
2. Shiver, Phil. The Blaze. Top medical journal may have to retract negative hydroxychloroquine conclusions after its study used suspect data. Published June 3, 2020. https://www.theblaze.com/news/top-medical-journal-suspect-data-hydroxychloroquine
3. Durden, Tyler. ZeroHedge.com. Massive WHO study Remdesivir doesn't lower COVID-19 mortality. Published October 15, 2020. https://www.zerohedge.com/geopolitical/massive-who-study-shows-remdesivir-doesnt-lower-covid-19-mortality
4. Durden, Tyler. ZeroHedge.com. WHO officially counsels against prescribing Gilead's Remdesivir to treat COVID-19. Published November 19, 2020. https://www.zerohedge.com/geopolitical/who-officially-counsels-against-prescribing-gileads-remdesivir-covid
5. Durden, Tyler. ZeroHedge.com. Collateral damage? CDC admits COVID lockdowns sparked surge in children's mental health issues. Published November 14, 2020. https://www.zerohedge.com/medical/collateral-damage-cdc-admits-covid-lockdowns-sparked-surge-childrens-mental-health-issues

6. This tweet has disappeared now, as far as I can tell. Evidence of its existence has been buried.
7. Chronicles Health. Published September 5, 2020. https://www.chronicleshealth.com/children/depressio n-rate-in-the-united-states-triples-during-covid-pandemic-research-shows/
8. Miltimore, John. FEE.org. 'A year's worth of suicide attempts in four weeks': the unintended consequences of COVID-19 lockdowns. Published May 26, 2020. https://fee.org/articles/a-years-worth-of-suicide-attempts-in-four-weeks-the-unintended-consequences-of-covid-19-lockdowns/
9. Widburg, Andrea. AmericanThinker.com. Now the World Health Organization is meddling with our teeth. Published August 14, 2020. https://www.americanthinker.com/blog/2020/08/no w_the_world_health_organization_is_meddling_with _our_teeth.html
10. Durden, Tyler. ZeroHedge.com. Health experts call for suspension of Pfizer vaccination among elderly after Norway deaths. Published January 16, 2021. https://www.zerohedge.com/covid-19/norway-sounds-alarm-over-vaccine-risks-elderly-frail-after-23-deaths
11. I have catalogued these videos extensively on Telegram @Aden Tate is Writing.
12. Snyder, Michael. ZeroHedge.com. UN World Food Program warns of "famines of Biblical proportions in 2021". Published November 19, 2020. https://www.zerohedge.com/geopolitical/un-world-food-program-warns-famines-biblical-proportions-2021

Chapter 11

1. Sovereign Man. Jellyfish News. To save people from COVID, Puerto Rico shuts down 911 call. Centers. Published October 24, 2020.

https://johnbwellsnews.com/to-save-people-from-covid-puerto-rico-shuts-down-911-call-centers/

2. Sacca, Paul. The Blaze. California to release 8000 inmates in attempt to combat COVID-19 spike in prisons. Published July 11, 2020. https://www.theblaze.com/news/california-release-8-000-prisoners

3. Durden, Tyler. ZeroHedge.com. San Francisco orders new COVID lockdown; CDC asks Americans to wear masks indoors unless at home. Published December 4, 2020. https://www.zerohedge.com/geopolitical/more-10-states-see-record-covid-numbers-china-says-600mm-vaccine-doses-ready-go-live

4. Durden, Tyler. ZeroHedge.com. Mayor Garcetti bans walking as latest LA lockdown begins. Published December 4, 2020. https://www.zerohedge.com/political/mayor-garcetti-bans-walking-latest-la-lockdown-begins

Chapter 12

1. Widburg, Andrea. AmericanThinker.com. Cornell exempts non-white students from its flu vaccine requirement. Published December 9, 2020. https://www.americanthinker.com/blog/2020/12/cornell_exempts_nonwhite_students_from_its_flu_vaccine_requirement.html

2. OffGridSurvival.com. Oregon county issues face mask order that exempts non-white people. Published June 23, 2020. https://offgridsurvival.com/oregon-county-issues-face-mask-order-that-exempts-non-white-people/

3. Sacca, Paul. The Blaze. Two US cities declare racism a public health emergency. Published July 18, 2020. https://www.theblaze.com/news/racism-public-health-emergency-minneapolis

4. Garcia, Carlos. The Blaze. NYC Mayor de Blasio says he's banning all large gatherings to stop coronavirus – except

for BLM protests. Published July 9, 2020. https://www.theblaze.com/news/deblasio-ban-blm-coronavirus-gathering

5. Enloe, Chris. The Blaze. All-Democrat city council revokes business license of gym that refuses to remain shut down. Published August 12, 2020. https://www.theblaze.com/news/all-democrat-city-council-revokes-business-license-from-gym-that-refused-to-remain-shut-down

6. Durden, Tyler. ZeroHedge.com. Cuomo delays release of data on New York's COVID-19 deaths until after election. Published September 2, 2020. https://www.zerohedge.com/political/cuomo-struggles-delay-release-data-new-yorks-covid-19-nursing-home-deaths

7. Durden, Tyler. Lori Lightfoot tells Chicago: cancel Thanksgiving, avoid family, days after hosting crowded Biden street party. Published November 14, 2020. https://www.zerohedge.com/political/lori-lightfoot-tells-chicago-cancel-thanksgiving-avoid-family-days-after-hosting-crowded

8. OffGridSurvival.com. Cuomo and Democrat governors to block vaccine until Biden is in as president. Published November 9, 2020. https://offgridsurvival.com/cuomo-and-dem-governors-to-block-vaccine-until-biden-in-as-president/

9. Widburg, Andrea. ZeroHedge.com. LA County's public health director accidentally admits what many suspected about lockdowns. Published September 11, 2020. https://www.zerohedge.com/political/la-countys-public-health-director-accidentally-admits-what-many-suspected-about-lockdowns

10. Durden, Tyler. ZeroHedge.com. Suddenly optimistic Fauci sees pandemic "plateauing" , fells "liberated" under Biden admin. Published January 21, 2020. https://www.zerohedge.com/covid-19/us-covid-

hospitalizations-reach-turning-point-dr-fauci-
confirms-joining-whos-gates-backed

11. Colen, Aaron. The Blaze. Wisconsin state employees
    required to wear masks even when they're home in
    virtual meetings. Published August 12, 2020.
    https://www.theblaze.com/news/wisconsin-state-
    employees-masks-zoom

12. Colen, Aaron. The Blaze. Los Angeles County escalates
    COVID-19 lockdown battle with John MacArthur's
    church by terminating parking lot lease. Published
    September 1, 2020.
    https://www.theblaze.com/news/la-county-john-
    macarthur-church-parking-lot

13. Urbanski, Dave. The Blaze. Church cited after maskless
    pastor - who's alone in building – answers the door for
    health official. Warnings of closure, fines, jail time
    follow. Published December 2, 2020.
    https://www.theblaze.com/news/church-cited-
    maskless-pastor-alone-in-building--answers-door-for-
    health-official-warnings-of-closure-fines-jail-time-
    follow

14. Horowitz, Daniel. NYC officials target Jewish business
    owner for COVID citation, while Biden supporters hold
    wild parties. Published November 9, 2020.
    https://www.theblaze.com/op-ed/ready-horowitz-nyc-
    officials-target-jewish-business-owner-for-covid-
    citation-while-biden-supporters-hold-wild-parties

15. Durden, Tyler. ActivistPost.com. New York sends "mask
    squads" to enforce social distancing in two counties.
    Published December 8, 2020.
    https://www.activistpost.com/2020/12/new-york-
    sends-mask-squads-to-enforce-social-distancing-in-
    two-counties.html

16. Field, Chris. The Blaze. NYC Mayor de Blasio fines
    synagogue $15K for massive secret wedding, says house
    of worship will be closed down if there's 'any further
    illegal activity'. Published November 24, 2020.

https://www.theblaze.com/news/de-blasio-punishes-synagogue-massive-secret-wedding

17. Field, Chris. The Blaze. Dozens of police barricade Canadian church parking lot to keep worshippers out of drive-in service. So they line the highway instead. Published December 1, 2020. https://www.theblaze.com/news/police-barricade-church-parking-lot

18. Adams, Samuel. *The Rights of the Colonists as Men.*

Chapter 13

1. PewPewTactical.com. Guns sales pre and post COVID: what the numbers are saying. Published 2020. https://www.pewpewtactical.com/guns-sales-pre-post-covid/

2. Durden, Tyler. ZeroHedge.com. De Blasio's New York: bulletproof vest sales are skyrocketing in parts of the city. Published August 16, 2020. https://www.zerohedge.com/political/de-blasios-new-york-bulletproof-vest-sales-are-skyrocketing-parts-city

3. Durden, Tyler. ZeroHedge.com. GW University reports 17% enrollment drop as students opt out of COVID-restricted campus life. Published September 15, 2020. https://www.zerohedge.com/economics/gw-university-reports-17-enrollment-drop-students-opt-out-covid-restricted-campus-life

4. Pandolfo, Chris. The Blaze. South Dakota gov. Kristi Noem won't comply if Biden pursues national mask mandate. Published November 13, 2020. https://www.theblaze.com/news/kristi-noem-will-not-comply-biden-mask-mandate

5. Enloe, Chris. The Blaze. New York sheriff takes defiant stance against gov. Cuomo's COVID restrictions impacting Thanksgiving. Published November 16, 2020. https://www.theblaze.com/news/new-york-sheriff-defiant-cuomo-covid-thanksgiving

6. Utter, Eric. AmericanThinker.com. New York gov. Cuomo says that his word is law, bands gatherings of more than 10 people just in time for Thanksgiving. Published November 22, 2020. https://www.americanthinker.com/blog/2020/11/new _york_gov_cuomo_says_that_his_word_is_law_bans _gatherings_of_more_than_10_people_just_in_time _for_thanksgiving.html
7. Durden, Tyler. ZeroHedge.com. 'Le Grand Escape' from Paris: footage shows record-breaking traffic gridlock hours before lockdown. Published November 1, 2020. https://www.zerohedge.com/political/le-grand-escape-paris-lockdown-stunning-footage-shows-highway-gridlock-miles

Chapter 14

1. Bastiat, Frederic. *The Law*. Tribeca Books. Auburn, AL. 2007. Pg. 23-24.
2. Frank, BN. ActivistPost.com. 750 million genetically engineered mosquitoes are being released in Florida despite environmental opposition. Published August 20, 2020. https://www.activistpost.com/2020/08/750-million-genetically-engineered-mosquitoes-are-being-released-in-florida-despite-environmental-opposition.html
3. Taylor, Sarah. The Blaze. Florida government to release 750 million genetically engineered mosquitoes in unique experiment. Published August 21, 2020. https://www.theblaze.com/news/florida-government-genetically-engineered-mosquitoes

Chapter 15

1. Bastiat, Frederic. *The Law*. Tribeca Books. Auburn, AL. 2007. Pg. 22-23.
2. Rand, Ayn. *Capitalism: The Unknown Ideal*. New American Library. New York, New York. 1966. Pg. 332.

3. Darrah, Nicole. Fox News. Hawaii police officer pleads guilty to forcing man to lick public urinal to avoid arrest. Published December 18, 2019. https://www.foxnews.com/us/hawaii-forces-man-to-lick-urinal

4. Lloyd, Novick. *Public Health Administration: Principles for Population-Based Management.* Jones and Bartlett Learning. 2007. Pg. 135.

5. Taylor, Sarah. The Blaze. Ohio lawmakers say elective medical procedures could be postponed amid 'exponential' surge in COVID-19 cases. Published November 24, 2020. https://www.theblaze.com/news/ohio-lawmakers-say-elective-medical-procedures-could-be-postponed-amid-exponential-surge-in-covid-19-case

6. McCrystal, Laura. The Philadelphia Inquirer. A timeline of Philadelphia's soda tax. https://www.inquirer.com/news/timeline-philadelphias-soda-tax-20190429.html

7. Black, Simon. ActivistPost.com. You can now be fined, jailed and assaulted for not wearing a mask (and other tyrannical weekly news). Published July 31, 2020. https://www.activistpost.com/2020/07/fined-jailed-and-assaulted-for-not-wearing-a-mask-and-other-tyrannical-weekly-news.html

8. Whitehead, John. ActivistPost.com. Virtual school dangers: the hazards of a police state education during COVID-19. Published September 15, 2020. https://www.activistpost.com/2020/09/virtual-school-dangers-the-hazards-of-a-police-state-education-during-covid-19.html

9. Frank, BN. ActivistPost.com. Los Angeles authorizes shutting off utility services of homes hosting large gatherings. Published August 8, 2020. https://www.activistpost.com/2020/08/los-angeles-authorizes-shutting-off-utility-services-to-homes-hosting-large-gatherings.html

10. Adams, Samuel. *The Rights of the Colonists as Men*

11. Paine, Thomas. *Common Sense.*

Chapter 16

1. Mill, John Stuart. *On Liberty.* AHM Publishing Corporation. Arlington Heights, IL. 1947. Pg. 12-13.

Chapter 17

1. Urbanski, Dave. The Blaze. Man arrested for allegedly threatening to shoot up yeshiva children's camp over lack of social distancing. Published August 19, 2020. https://www.theblaze.com/news/man-arrested-yeshiva-camp-threats
2. OffGridSurvival.com. New York scares the s out of public: turns Empire State Building into dystopian emergency siren. Published March 31, 2020. https://offgridsurvival.com/empire-state-building-into-dystopian-emergency-siren/
3. Dumas, Breck. The Blaze. 'It's a disgrace': father left heartbroken after Disney World refused entry to disabled daughter who cannot wear a mask. Published August 17, 2020. https://www.theblaze.com/news/father-heartbroken-after-disney-refused-entry-to-disabled-daughter-who-cannot-wear-mask

Chapter 18

1. Betts, Stephen. The Courier. Sheriff's office investigates felled-tree incident on Vinalhaven. Published March 29, 2020. https://www.pressherald.com/2020/03/29/sheriffs-office-issues-notice-following-felled-tree-incident-on-vinalhaven/
2. Price, Mark. The News and Observer. Outer Banks blocking roads, refusing to allow outsiders amid coronavirus outbreak. Published July 15, 2020.

https://www.newsobserver.com/news/coronavirus/art
icle241265921.html

Chapter 19

1. Hayek, FA. The Road to Serfdom. The University of
   Chicago Press. Routledge, London. 2007. Pg. 152.
2. The Burning Platform. "That mask is giving you lung
   cancer" Becky Ayers. Published October 24, 2020.
   https://www.theburningplatform.com/2020/10/24/th
   at-mask-is-giving-you-lung-cancer-becky-
   akers/#more-226930
3. Watson, Paul. ZeroHedge.com. Maine governor orders
   restaurant staff to wear COVID-visors like dog-cones.
   Published   August   20,   2020.
   https://www.zerohedge.com/political/maine-
   governor-orders-restaurant-staff-wear-covid-visors-
   dog-cones
4. Whitehead, John. ActivistPost.com. Virtual school
   dangers: the hazards of a police state education during
   COVID-19.   Published   September   15,   2020.
   https://www.activistpost.com/2020/09/virtual-
   school-dangers-the-hazards-of-a-police-state-
   education-during-covid-19.html
5. Garcia, Carlos. The Blaze. Customer calls out Starbucks
   employee for refusing service over mask – then the
   internet steps in with a $22k payday. Published June 25,
   2020.   https://www.theblaze.com/news/starbucks-
   mask-san-diego-refusal
6. Horowitz, Daniel. The Blaze. CDC study: 85% of COVID-
   19 cases in July were people who often or always wear
   masks.   Published   October   12,   2020.
   https://www.theblaze.com/op-ed/horowitz-cdc-study-
   covid-masks
7. Horowitz, Daniel. The Blaze. From Fort Benning to
   Japan and Hawaii, face masks are not working.
   Published   August   3,   2020.
   https://www.theblaze.com/horowitz-from-fort-

benning-to-japan-and-hawaii-face-masks-are-not-working

8. Rand, Ayn. *Capitalism: The Unknown Ideal.* New American Library. New York, NY. 1966. Pg. 173.

9. Miltimore, John. ZeroHedge.com. World's top epidemiologists – masks don't work!. Published August 8, 2020. https://www.zerohedge.com/political/worlds-top-epidemiologists-masks-dont-work

10. Watson, Steve. ZeroHedge.com. Sweden's lead epidemiologist: wearing face masks is "very dangerous". Published August 21, 2020. https://www.zerohedge.com/medical/swedens-lead-epidemiologist-wearing-face-masks-very-dangerous

11. Hounsell, Scott. RedState.com. The CDC accidentally admits cloth masks are not effective. Published September 10, 2020. https://www.redstate.com/scotthounsell/2020/09/10/the-cdc-accidentally-admits-cloth-masks-are-not-effective/

12. Horowitz, Daniel. The Blaze. CDChttps://www.theblaze.com/op-ed/horowitz-cdc-study-covid-masks

13. Principia Scientifica. Study shows how mask wearing INCREASES infection risk! Published March 24, 2021. https://principia-scientific.com/contamination-by-respiratory-viruses-on-outer-surface-of-medical-masks/

14. Rand. *Capitalism.* Pg. 325.

Chapter 20

1. OffGridSurvival.com. And it begins! New York to require mandatory COVID-19 testing for out-of-state travelers. Published October 31, 2020. https://offgridsurvival.com/and-it-begins-new-york-to-require-mandatory-covid-19-testing-for-out-of-state-travelers/

2. Mill, John Stuart. *On Liberty*. AHM Publishing Corporation. Arlington Heights, IL. 1947. Pg. 97.

Chapter 23

1. Rand, Ayn. *Capitalism: The Unknown Ideal*. New World Books. New York, NY. 1966. Pg. 325.
2. Ibid., Pg. 324.

Chapter 24

1. Mill, John Stuart. *On Liberty*. AHM Publishing Corporation. Arlington Heights, IL. 1947. Pg. 12.
2. *Ibid.* p14
3. Hayek, FA. *The Road to Serfdom*. The University of Chicago Press. Routledge, London. 2007. Pg. 176.
4. Piper, Jessica. Maine Public. Maine suspends Waterville doctor's license for alleged COVID-19 misinformation. Published November 29, 2021. https://www.mainepublic.org/health/2021-11-29/maine-suspends-waterville-doctors-license-for-alleged-covid-19-misinformation
5. Hayek. Pg. 171.
6. Paul, Rand. *The Case Against Socialism*. HarperCollins Publishers. New York, NY. 2019. Pg 214.
7. Mill. Pg. 17.
8. Hayek. Pg. 175.
9. Orwell, George. *Animal Farm*. New American Library. New York, NY. 1996. Pg. 88.

Chapter 25

1. Rand, Ayn. *Capitalism: The Unknown Ideal*. New World Books. New York, NY. 1966. Pg. 320.
2. Rand, Ayn. *Anthem*. New American Library. New York, NY. 1995. Pg. 16.
3. Paul, Rand. *The Case Against Socialism*. HarperCollins Publishers. New York, NY. 2019. Pg 17-18.

4. *Ibid.* Pg. 14.
5. *Ibid.* Pg. 15.
6. *Ibid.* Pg. 2-3.
7. *Ibid.* Pg. 16.
8. *Ibid.* Pg. 28.

Chapter 26

1. Paul, Rand. *The Case Against Socialism.* HarperCollins Publishers. New York, NY. 2019. Pg 5.
2. Hayek, FA. *The Road to Serfdom.* The University of Chicago Press. Routledge, London. 2007. Pg. 168.
3. Ibid., Pg. 169.
4. Paul, Rand. Pg. 52.
5. Hayek, FA. Pg. 170.
6. Ibid., Pg. 67.
7. Ibid., Pg. 79.

Chapter 27

1. Freedland, Jonathan. The Guardian. Eugenics: The skeleton that rattles loudest in the left's closet. Published February 17, 2012. https://www.theguardian.com/commentisfree/2012/feb/17/eugenics-skeleton-rattles-loudest-closet-left
2. Rand, Ayn. *Capitalism: The Unknown Ideal.* Signet Printing. New York, NY. 1967. Pg. 23-24.
3. Paul, Rand. *The Case Against Socialism.* HarperCollins Publishers. New York, NY. 2019. Pg 156-157.
4. Ibid., Pg. 158.

Chapter 28

1. Barnes & Noble. *The Constitution of the United States of America: And Selected Writings of the Founding Fathers.* Barnes & Noble. New York, NY. 2012. Pg. 140.
2. Hayek, FA. *The Road to Serfdom.* The University of Chicago Press. Routledge, London. 2007. Pg. 153.

3. Barnes & Noble. Pg. 152.
4. Orwell, George. *Animal Farm*. New American Library. New York, NY. 1996. Pg. 35.
5. *Ibid*. Pg. 53.

Chapter 29

1. Rand, Ayn. *Anthem*. New American Library. New York, NY. 1995. Pg. 15-16.
2. Hayek, FA. *The Road to Serfdom*. The University of Chicago Press. Routledge, London. 2007. Pg. 140.

Chapter 30

1. Pickover, Clifford. *The Medical Book*. Union Square and Co. 2012. Page 370
2. Ibid. pg. 324
3. The Daily Expose. Pfizer document confirms concerns of 'vaccine shedding' after thousands of women report irregular bleeding and miscarriage. Published May 17, 2021. https://dailyexpose.uk/2021/05/17/pfizer-document-confirms-concerns-of-vaccine-shedding-after-thousands-of-women-report-irregular-bleeding-and-miscarriage/

Afterword

1. Hayek, FA. *The Road to Serfdom*. The University of Chicago Press. Routledge, London. 2007. Pg. 210.
2. Rand, Ayn. *Capitalism: The Unknown Ideal*. Signet Printing. New York, NY. 1967. Pg. 182.
3. Ibid., Pg. 147.
4. Ibid., Pg. 149
5. Paine, Thomas. *The Crisis*. Penguin Books. New York, NY. 1995.
6. Ibid.
7. Ibid.
8. Ibid.

References

9. Rawles, James Wesley. *Patriots: A Novel of Survival in the Coming Collapse*. Ulysses Press. Berkeley, CA. 2013. Pg. 324.

Other Books by Blacksmith Publishing

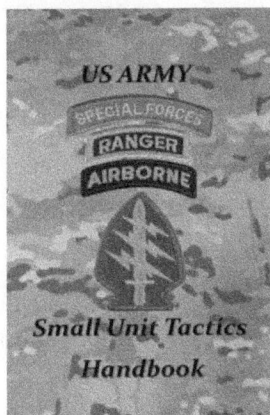

Small Unit Tactics Handbook

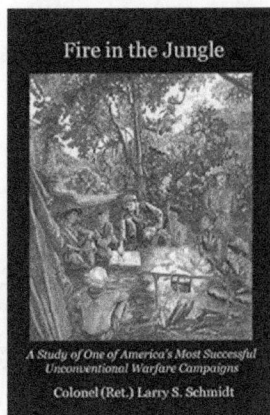

Fire in the Jungle

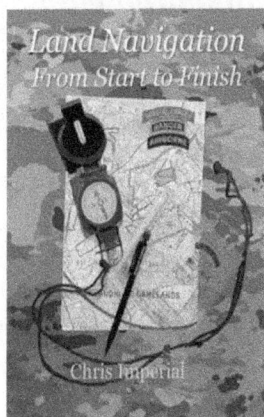

Land Navigation From Start to Finish

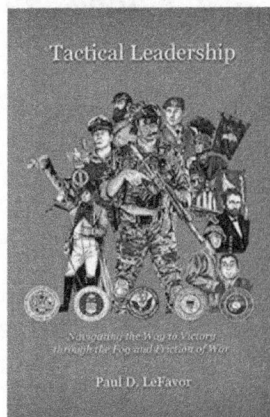

Tactical Leadership

www.blacksmithpublishing.com

www.ingramcontent.com/pod-product-compliance
Lightning Source LLC
Chambersburg PA
CBHW022043020426
42335CB00012B/519